Yoga
Turns Back the Clock

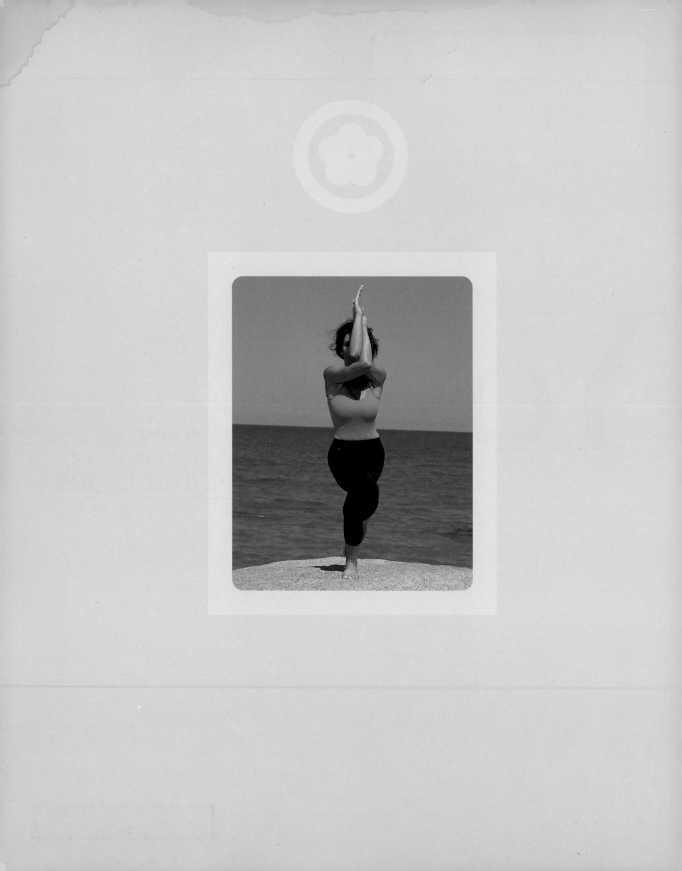

GLENDA TWINING

WITH MARK SEAL

FOREWORD BY JORGE CRUISE

Yoga
Turns Back the Clock

THE UNIQUE

TOTAL-BODY PROGRAM

THAT FIGHTS FAT,

WRINKLES, AND FATIGUE

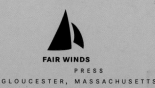

FAIR WINDS
PRESS
GLOUCESTER, MASSACHUSETTS

Text © 2003 by Glenda Twining
Photographs © 2003 by Fair Winds Press

First published in the USA in 2003 by
Fair Winds Press
33 Commercial Street
Gloucester, MA 01930

Library of Congress Cataloging-in-Publication data available

ISBN 1-59233-006-1

10 9 8 7 6 5 4 3 2 1

Cover design by Mary Ann Smith Design
Book design by Yee Design
Photography by Bobbie Bush Photography. www.bobbiebush.com

Printed and bound in China

The information in this book is for educational purposes only. It is not intended to
replace the advice of a physician or medical practitioner. Please see your health care
provider before beginning any new health program.

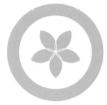

contents

FOREWORD

Hi! I'm Jorge Cruise, the author of the *New York Times* best-selling book *8 Minutes in the Morning: A Simple Way to Shed Up to 2 Pounds a Week Guaranteed* (HarperCollins). I want to congratulate you for taking the first step to getting in shape and restoring your youthful appearance—the natural way. In a time when Botox injections, liposuction, and fad diet pills are accessible to the masses, it's encouraging to see people turning to exercise—instead of the quick fix—to make them feel *and look* better!

Many of us are tempted to think that we are too old to start an exercise routine, but nothing could be further from the truth. If you decide to embark on a new path that includes exercise, yoga is the ideal choice. Besides slowing the signs of aging, yoga can give you more energy, a tighter body, and a more positive outlook than you've had in years. Bottom line: Exercise CAN make you feel young. More specifically, yoga with Glenda Twining can transform your life!

I was in Dallas recently with my literary agent, working on my next book, *8 Minutes in the Morning for Real Shape, Real Size: A Simple Way to Shed 30 Pounds or More* (Rodale), when he convinced me to go to a class hosted by a woman he calls the Yoga Goddess, Glenda Twining. I took her workshop and I was amazed at how rejuvenated I felt inside and out when I finished. This isn't just any ordinary yoga program. Having been a figure in the fitness world for years, I have taken every kind of exercise class available, and none have left me as satisfied and energized as Glenda's. Her extraordinary age-erasing yoga will open your eyes to the power of exercise on your figure and your psyche! Glenda is the proof that these routines work—at 50 years old, she doesn't look a day over 35. She has achieved this through discipline and by faithfully practicing her special brand of yoga.

Glenda will leave you stretched, toned, and feeling a tranquility you can only achieve through yoga. By following her routine, you will lose weight and stretch your muscles for a more toned body; but the benefits extend beyond fitness! Glenda's yoga routine can keep your skin and hair healthy and can help keep you looking young. When you look at Glenda you see a timeless woman who swears the way to stay young is through her program. And she is right! The amazing thing is you *will* finish her routine feeling and looking younger. I have never been to class that did more for the mind, body, and appearance.

I was so happy to hear that Glenda was going to share her secrets with the world through this wonderful book. I know you will find the same great results and satisfaction I found after meeting Glenda. Enjoy, and feel great!

Jorge Cruise

America's #1 online weight-loss specialist with more than 3 million clients

www.jorgecruise.com

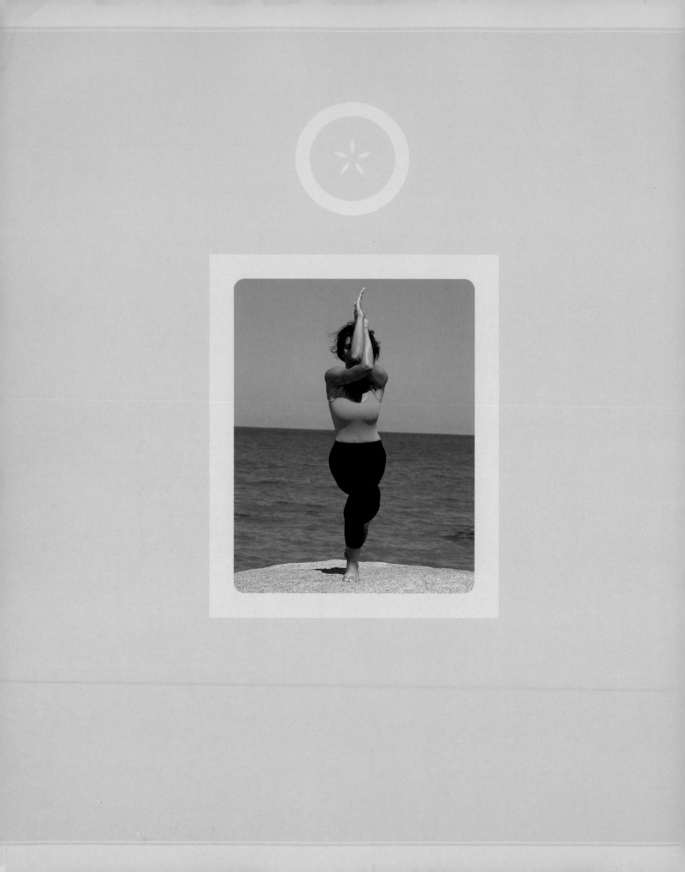

Chapter 1

How to Stop the Aging Clock

There is a fountain of youth, and it awaits you. It's not in a forest or hidden on some magic mountain—it's a fountain that exists within you. To unleash it, all you have to do is follow the program detailed in this book.

It's a program built on yoga, but yoga is only the beginning.

It's a program that can lead you through a dramatic transformation. Not only will you feel more youthful, more energized, and more alive, you will also actually turn back the aging clock.

Let's start with the yoga part of the program. Then we'll get to the magic.

The International Association of Yoga Therapists groups the benefits of yoga into three categories: physiological benefits, psychological benefits, and biochemical benefits. Among the reported benefits of routine yoga practice is something of a recipe for eternal youth:

Increased cardiovascular efficiency
Decreased blood pressure
Improved posture
Increased immunity
Decreased hostility and depression
Improved balance
Improved memory and concentration
Decreased cholesterol

Endless studies have been conducted to quantify the benefits of yoga. The April 23, 2001, issue of *Time* magazine reported a study by Dr. Dean Ornish on patients with coronary heart disease. Dr. Ornish discovered that a "regimen of aerobic exercise and stress reduction, including yoga, combined with a low-fat vegetarian diet, stabilized and in some cases reversed arterial blockage."

The program you hold in your hands performs a similar feat, taking traditional yoga to a new and even more energizing level where it not only halts the stages of aging, but actually turns back the aging clock.

I have seen the magic of yoga work, and not merely through the amazing results experienced by my students. I've also experienced these results firsthand.

At 50, I am my own best testimonial. Practicing every class with my students—eleven packed, back-to-back group classes and nine privates each week—I've suffered no injuries, even though I constantly test my limits. I am strong, flexible, toned, focused, calm, and hormonally balanced. At an age when I should be experiencing full menopausal symptoms, practicing yoga consistently has kept me from suffering any effects at all of what is sometimes defined as a "disabling process." On the contrary, I have never felt better or more energized.

I was always petite, but I never had toned or well-defined muscles. Since beginning this program, though, I've replaced fat with muscle. My body has become totally toned and supple. My friends and clients continue to be amazed by my youthful appearance, and they're even more shocked when they see the results they achieve for themselves.

Five years ago, my body fat was 20 percent; now it hovers around 11 to 13 percent. I used to get bladder infections, but I haven't had one in five years, thanks to the yoga poses that massage the bladder and urinary tract. I constantly feel energetic and emotionally uplifted. I've recently remarried, and I have a wonderful, supportive, and loving husband, as well as a host of exciting new projects in the pipeline.

In the midst of what could be a very stressful situation, though, I am consistently calm and centered, with none of the irritability or anxiousness that I used to feel as a result of stress. This is due to the natural stress-busting attributes of yoga. I have a youthful appearance that emanates from within. I have a spring in my step. I am focused and feel very balanced, and I'm very appreciative of life and the wonderful gift of this miraculous body and mind I possess.

Yoga has been a gift, practically a gift of eternal youth, and I want to share it with you. This book, if followed regularly, will be just as beneficial as attending my classes on a regular basis.

Youthfulness emanates from the energy within us. Whether you are 16 or 76, I can help you restore and rekindle that energy. I believe in this program so much that it has become my lifestyle. This book is designed to become a diary that you can keep with you, a book that provides support, instruction, inspiration, and motivation throughout your entire transformation. Followed consistently, this workout yields age-shattering results for clients of any age group or fitness level. It's a beautiful experience with health-giving effects that will find their way into every aspect of your life.

DID YOU KNOW?

The secret to halting, then reversing, the aging process is in the spine.

The health and flexibility of your spine dictates your overall health and beauty. The spine is the supporting structure and command center for the nerves stretching throughout your entire body. A flexible, strong, aligned, healthy spine emanates youthfulness. Poor posture—a hunched upper back coupled with a swayed lower back—will make you feel and look old. Sitting at a desk or computer, and even the everyday routine of driving, allows gravity to compact the spine. Nonstop movement, coupled with my program's balanced yoga postures, will move the spine effectively to counteract gravity. The result will be increased mobility and suppleness.

If you are already exercising—jogging, swimming, or maybe weight lifting—yoga is a wonderful addition to your regimen. This is because while other activities exercise only a few areas, yoga, and this program specifically, is designed for a total workout. It exercises your joints, and stretches and massages all your internal organs, your muscles, your tendons, your nervous system and, most importantly, your spine.

Why is this important? To begin with, most people suffer from a very early age with low back problems that could easily be eliminated by keeping a supple spine. Also, if you are into any sport, from golf to soccer, you most likely repeatedly use one side of the body. This can cause a strain on and weakness in your other limbs and spine, leading to an imbalance or weakness in certain areas of your body. One side becomes more flexible and stronger, and the lack of balance between the left and right sides of your body affects the spine and—in most cases—causes chronic pain.

When balance is achieved, all systems work perfectly. Our bodies were not designed to move in just one dimension, pattern, or direction. Doing so is like setting out a welcome mat for premature aging. Your body is extremely resilient, though; it's capable of recapturing youth and vitality at any age. Bone density and structure can change, and ligaments, tendons, and muscles can become limber and stretch out.

Yoga can shift you from being stiff and rigid, in both mind and body, to being strong, flexible, and well balanced. You will be changing your entire body, internally and externally, mentally and physically. You will feel a total change in your happiness and outlook on life.

After your first session of Routine 1, you will immediately feel a shift in your spine, and then a bigger shift as your body's suppleness improves. This feeling will prepare you for the next workout session, which will move your progress to yet another level. This constant feeling of improvement will keep you totally inspired and motivated to continue. The overall benefit is that you will start to regain suppleness in your spine and balance in your life.

THE DISCOVERY OF AGE-DEFYING YOGA

In my adopted hometown of Dallas, Texas, I was a successful conventional physical fitness trainer for many years. I have employed traditional weight training techniques for two vastly different specialties: preparing mountain climbers for their greatest challenges, and helping extremely overweight women lose pounds and get in shape. As a fitness trainer, my results were definitely acceptable, even sought-after, but I wanted something more.

I wanted something age-shattering, a program that could actually stop, then reverse, the aging process.

When I was 45, I stumbled upon yoga. Always seeking new ways to maximize my fitness-training program, I began thinking about yoga. I bought a Yoga Journal magazine, ordered some "Power Yoga" tapes, and began practicing. When I felt immediate results, I wanted to do more.

After a period of study, I went to my birthplace, Johannesburg, South Africa, and studied under a noted yoga guru for three intensive months, practicing eight hours each day. I discovered that the practice of yoga not only increases flexibility and strength, it also dramatically improves the body's hormonal balance. This translates into greater inner peace and mental stability. I instantly knew that yoga was the direction I needed to follow in both my life and my career, so I gave up my work as a fitness specialist to devote myself exclusively to yoga.

I began studying every style of yoga I could find. I received my certificate from the Houston Institute of Yoga, then directed by Lex Gillian, who runs wonderfully intensive teachers' training courses, including training in meditation.

Then, I met the legendary Baron Baptiste, who teaches throughout America and internationally, as well. He was brought up in a family of yoga practitioners and is one of the country's leading teachers. I learned much from Baron and assisted in hosting seventy students at two of his yoga retreats in the Yucatan.

I watched yoga change the lives of my own clients with its many beneficial qualities. I had found success once again, this time as a yoga instructor. And once again, my results were great, but not enough.

It still wasn't age-shattering.

Back in Dallas, I heard that a prominent Dallas chiropractor was seeking a yoga instructor for his practice. He had interviewed more than twenty-five instructors before me. I got the position, which turned out to be a gift. The classes started small: I had only four students the first time I taught at the clinic. We moved the chiropractic beds off the floor to make space, and I held the sessions right in the middle of the cramped room.

The chiropractor put a microphone with a headpiece over my head, but it kept falling off and it restricted many movements. I had to teach the class from a corner of the room, which made it hard for people to really see me. Still, the response was great and everyone was so supportive. Within two months I had twenty-six people flooding this tiny, carpeted, elongated room that we had to spend a good half-hour moving furniture around every time I taught a class!

Between classes, I still trained individual athletes and less active students at a ballroom dance studio. Because the studio was empty during the day, the management let me have it for practically nothing. There was nothing but four walls, a parquet floor, and a stereo, but that was all I needed to jump-start my revolution in fitness training. During the first class, I had some really exotic yoga music on the stereo and was joined by a few of the people who worked at the ballroom. We all got on the floor and started practicing the yoga moves.

The beat of the music was fast, and I started to move at a little quicker pace and add some of my fitness training into the yoga postures. Everyone started to sweat and enjoy the momentum. I would begin in a yoga posture and end in a sculpting move that took nothing away from the posture, but instead enhanced it. One pose segued into the other, until we were working out for practically an hour without stopping.

When we ended the session, we all looked at each other, hearts pumping, wet with sweat, but absolutely limber and energized.

It was the best workout, ever.

That's when it hit me that I could combine the nutritional and toning benefits of traditional Western fitness training with the flexibility, strength, and mind-body benefits of yoga. Then, I would add a third, explosive ingredient: nonstop movement, from posture to posture. I had finally found a way to stop the aging clock.

My standard yoga sessions were already filled with beneficial techniques: relaxed, controlled breathing; an enhanced mind-body connection; balance;

flexibility and movement of the spine; and mental focus. But with my new awakening to the power of nonstop movement, my yoga sessions became revitalized. I found that by linking the poses to one another and eliminating stops between them, I could greatly increase the beneficial effects of each yoga session.

I began to infuse my yoga sessions with the most valuable of my physical fitness techniques: better living habits; positive, lifelong changes to eating routines; endurance training through gentle strength-building postures; and enhanced, nonstop movement of the entire body.

The next day, I walked into class at the chiropractor's office reborn. I started incorporating the fitness and aerobic elements and nonstop movement into the traditional yoga postures, just like I'd done in the ballroom. But I also added some abdominal exercises (strong stomach muscles are an absolute must for patients with back problems). The program deepened and got more intense.

I immediately saw tremendous results in both the chiropractic patients and the students attending classes. They all reported back how energetic they were feeling, how yoga was helping them move again without pain. They also gained flexibility and felt stronger.

Word spread fast about the little Dallas yoga class that could not only halt the aging process, but could actually turn back the aging clock. Without any advertising, my classes were soon packed to capacity in this cramped office space. We still had to move furniture for every class.

Prominent Dallas fitness guru Larry North hosts a radio show, has authored several fitness books, and runs gyms from Dallas to Miami. When he heard about my program, he invited me to open my own studio within his studio. Then, I was invited to teach at the Cooper Aerobics Center (owned and founded by the famed Kenneth Cooper), where the aerobics movement was born and continues to thrive. My classes at both venues are very well-supported by enthusiastic students and Cooper colleagues. The classes have been incredibly successful and always packed for one simple reason: The program works.

The secret to the success of this program is that I start you off with a yoga posture that transitions into a fitness move, and I continue to build on this foundation until you have mastered a variety of yoga and fitness pairings. The combination of yoga positions and fitness movements tones and sculpts your muscles. At the same time, all your major muscle groups experience a fat- and calorie-burning cardiovascular workout. The combination is very healthy for your heart when performed during an exercise routine that is low-impact and executed in a controlled manner. This program is designed for both athletes and nonathletes who want to develop strength, endurance, flexibility, and focus.

To begin seeing results, you'll need to practice at least three times a week for at least 30 minutes. At a later point, you may even want to work out more frequently or for longer periods of time. Your results will be determined by how much you give your workouts. Don't worry about having enough energy to expand your workout routine; the major benefit of this exercise combination is that it helps you become your own energy generator.

Even though I've run out of scheduling time to personally teach my Turning Back The Clock Workout, my courses continue to get more and more popular, and the waiting list for private clients gets longer and longer. So, to reach as many people as possible, I've put my techniques into a book.

WHAT YOGA CAN DO

Working with hundreds of people over the years, I've discovered that this combination of yoga practices and fitness exercises, along with some realistic nutritional changes, can help any individual reshape his or her body. By working with overweight women, athletes, and people of all ages, I have perfected this technique through constant evaluation of my clients' needs and results. In teaching large classes, sports teams, and individuals, I have come to fully understand how to get maximum results, as well as the secret to keeping people motivated.

Here are some of the things this powerhouse yoga workout will help you do:

1. *Achieve a balanced, youthful figure, whatever your age, and achieve self-awareness and mental clarity.*

2. *Rev up your metabolism for weight loss through postures that create an aerobic effect.*

3. *Tighten your muscles to build strength, then lengthen them to add flexibility, achieving a balanced approach to fitness.*

4. *Move your spine in every direction, giving you full flexibility and a young and supple spine. By opening the vertebrae and lengthening the spine with stretches, you'll avoid spinal degeneration.*

5. *Connect your mind and body. This results in greater mental focus, which will impact every area of your life. Your attention span will increase and, whatever your age, you will have greater focus and deeper concentration. In short, your brain will be more alert and youthful.*

6. *Build bone mass through yoga's natural resistance training, which utilizes your body's own weight, for the prevention or cure of osteoporosis.*

7. *Achieve a genuine sense of internal tranquility and peace. The calming effect of this will reduce anxiety and agitation, giving you an improved quality of life.*

8. *Build a healthier body by fueling it with the highest quality food. By forgetting the word diet and making a few changes, you will see the yoga program and nutritional changes help you achieve your goals.*

Making yoga a part of your lifestyle at any age is a sure way to increase your health and livelihood—and the benefits go way beyond appearances. You will have a renewed outlook on the world and your body that is derived from taking the steps to mindfully take care of yourself.

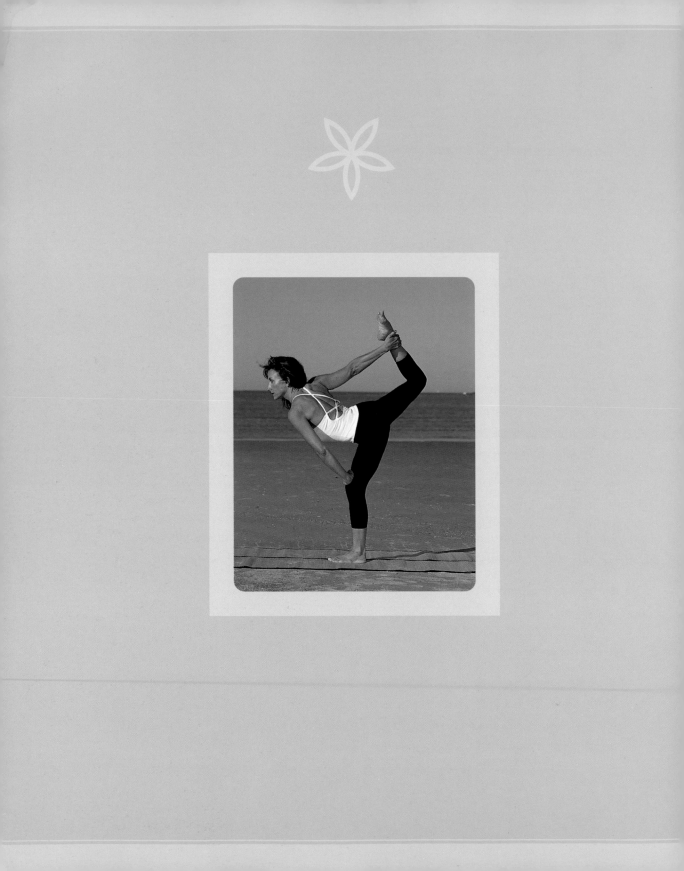

Chapter 2

The Magic of Movement

The first thing I tell my new students is, "Get moving!"

Most people think, "I'd be more active, if I had the energy," when the actual truth is that you'd have more energy if you were more active. Movement generates energy, and nonstop movement unleashes tremendous energy that can revitalize every area of your existence. It's impossible to achieve much in life without energy.

Lethargy increases the stresses of life, and stress is a major impediment to energy flow. Stress ages the mind, body, and spirit. Nonetheless, it's part of life. Our only option is not to fall victim to it. Only when we feel physically and mentally balanced are we best capable of dealing with stress. Yoga assists in developing a state of calm, strength, and confidence. The postures will help you accept and release stresses that come your way. So while you build a strong, flexible body, you will simultaneously build a strong, flexible mind. Yoga is a very healthy way to deal with stress.

The increased energy you feel will have a tremendous impact on your vitality and will help you gain the ultimate result: ageless, timeless beauty. It will help you look and feel healthy by increasing your metabolic rate.

WHY YOGA?

The practice of yoga began about 6,000 years ago. The name comes from a Sanskrit term meaning "the union of the body and mind." The most popular type of yoga, Hatha Yoga, actually means "yoga for health," combining the Sanskrit names ha (balance) and tha (moon). Hatha Yoga is centered in balance; its purpose is to join the different energy flows within the body. My program combines Hatha Yoga with three other major systems of ancient yoga.

BIKRAM

Named for Bikram Choudhury, the pioneer of this yoga system, Bikram Yoga distills ancient yoga into a sequence of twenty-six postures. Each posture is designed to enhance the functioning of every body system. Each pose is practiced twice, in a room heated to 100°F, to encourage sweating and the removal of impurities. Throughout, the ujjayi breath is used. This form of yoga is designed to encourage the cleansing of the body, the release of toxins, and maximum flexibility.

ASHTANGA

Ashtanga Yoga is a practice developed by Sri K. Pattabhi Jois, an Indian yoga master. His students brought the practice to America and elsewhere. The system is based on six series, each increasing in difficulty. Students learn the series of postures in a particular order, and the postures are linked together with connected movements to create a flowing sequence. The poses are linked by the deep breathing technique called the "ujjayi breath" and a flow of postures called vinyasas.

IYENGAR

Iyengar Yoga is a practice developed by B. K. S. Iyengar, an Indian master. This practice focuses on precise alignment and posture. The pace of the class is slower, and the poses are held for lengthy periods and repeated a few times each. This form of yoga is taught in stages: First, the standing poses are taught, with attention to the correct alignment of the feet, hips, pelvis, shoulders, and hands. Proper breathing is taught second. Many props are used—belts, blankets, bolsters, and so on—to help students achieve the best possible pose.

Throughout this book, I will show you how it is very possible to achieve your goals. This program is practical and easy to follow. It will require effort and dedication, but once you begin, you will reap obvious benefits.

To be successful at anything, whether it's a yoga session or some other facet of your life, you must grow in increments. Even if you only manage five minutes in the first session, that's a start. Set a goal to achieve ten minutes the next session. If you successfully complete the first session, go deeper in your poses and hold them a few breaths longer during the next session. You will gain self-discipline, determination, and concentration. The keys to success are patience and remembering that you are performing little miracles in your body day by day, session by session.

The process of aging is a gradual disintegration of the body and the mind. As we get older, we begin losing muscle tone; our muscles actually start shrinking, especially if we live a sedentary lifestyle. We lose our range of motion. Then, if we stay sedentary, we lose our ability to move at all.

As of this writing, regular exercise and a good diet are the main ways to stop this disabling process. Exercise is vitally important, as is stretching to promote flexibility and mobility in every part of your body. Working out with weights builds and firms your muscles, but muscle tone is just the beginning. To really turn back the clock, you must simultaneously train for flexibility and strength. Only yoga incorporates everything necessary to accomplish this.

As a bonus, yoga rejuvenates your endocrine system, which is made up of the glands that regulate hormonal secretions into the bloodstream and therefore determines our mood swings and emotions. The practice of yoga massages this system from the inside out, cleansing the glands and helping you avoid mood swings, depression, and anxiety.

How Yoga Stops the Aging Process

Aging can be traced to many sources. I discuss a few of the main ones below, preceded by testimonials from my clients describing how yoga has halted their aging process and put them on the road to a better, more fit, and more youthful life.

DEGENERATIVE SPINE

Due to a car accident, I developed degenerative spinal disc disease that affects my neck and lower back. Many types of exercise, such as weight lifting or running, aggravate my neck and lower back and cause me excruciating pain. It got to the point where I couldn't exercise at all and suffered pain constantly. I was losing muscle tone and couldn't even finish a cardiovascular workout. Glenda has helped me with her yoga routine. I started with private sessions and now attend her classes regularly. It's been wonderful for eliminating pain in both my neck and my back. I feel great and have improved my flexibility. I can move so much better. I am toned and am starting to get back to feeling normal again.

— LETITIA, 34

In yoga, there is an adage: "You are as young or old as your spine." Keeping your spine healthy is the most effective way to counteract the aging process. If we continually stretch and lengthen the spine for suppleness and flexibility, creating space between the vertebrae, the disks can return to a more youthful and healthy condition.

If you study a picture of the spine, you will notice there are four basic curves. There are two concave curves that dip into the body: one in the neck (cervcal), the other in the lower back (lumbar). Then, there are two convex curves that move away from the body: one in the tailbone (sacral); the other in the rib cage (thoracic). For the spine to be healthy, all four of these curves should be regularly stretched and exercised, creating equal spacing between the bones of the spine, the vertebrae.

The creation of space between the vertebrae is vital for the health of the spine, because this is how the nerves are released. When the spine is rigid and compressed from sitting and standing without stretching, the compressed vertebrae will pinch the nerves that pass through the vertebral cavity, causing pain and perhaps even muscular spasm. In acute cases, these pinched nerves may affect the health of organs and other body parts. Poor posture can cause digestion and other health problems if the flow of blood and the nerves leading to internal organs are restricted.

When we stretch and lengthen the spine, fluids are flushed in and out of and around the disks, keeping them nourished and healthy. Prolonged spinal inactivity and compression will cause the disks to shrink and lose their elasticity. Injuries, including herniated discs and pain from pressure, can result. Yoga prevents and corrects rounding of the spine and helps you regain spinal strength and flexibility.

BONE LOSS

I have been attending yoga with Glenda for about two years now and have never felt healthier. I have strength and flexibility and a sense of calmness. I would never have thought of yoga, but it certainly has changed my life. I recently went for a complete physical, especially to check for bone mass density and to see whether I was leaching calcium out of my bones, and the results were clear. "You have the bones of an 18-year-old," my doctor marveled. "Whatever you're doing, it's great."

— RAY, 50

Bones are strengthened primarily through weight-bearing exercise, which transmits signals to the bones that cause them to strengthen. Yoga is a superior form of weight-bearing exercise because it uses your body weight as resistance. To prevent bone loss and build a strong skeletal system, consistent practice of yoga is key.

Bones go through a constant state of loss and growth, with more loss than growth occurring as a person ages. Thin and fragile bones result in osteoporosis. This is an increased threat to women in their menopausal years, when the body produces less estrogen, the hormone that protects against bone loss.

To make matters worse, the common diet of soda and caffeine leaches minerals and calcium out of the bones. This poor diet, combined with little or no exercise, is an invitation to bone loss and a red carpet for premature aging. But this book will help you roll up that red carpet, because yoga combined with a correct diet builds bones.

Stress

I took Prozac for several years to treat depression and mild attention deficit disorder. But once I started taking Glenda's yoga classes consistently, I found that I didn't need Prozac any more. In addition, I reduced my weight training and cardio in the gym. I've found that I can maintain my strength and muscle tone with a reduced training schedule and still be much more flexible and relaxed.

—DEBORAH, 53

Stress is tremendously aging, and the way you react to a stressful situation is usually more harmful than the stressful event itself. Stress lowers your immune system and intensifies the aging process. And while we cannot entirely eliminate stressful events, we can change our emotional reactions through the practice of yoga positions, especially by observing the breath, staying in the moment, and quieting the mind. This allows the mind and body to become calmer and more balanced, while restoring equilibrium and recuperating from the stressful event.

For 6,000 years, yoga has served as the world's natural stress-buster. That's because the practice of yoga includes a powerful and deep relaxation technique. The deep, slow, rhythmic breathing incorporated into all yoga practices carries oxygen through your system and relaxes tense muscles. Many of the postures open and expand the chest, allowing you to breathe easier and more deeply, which has a calming effect.

As mentioned earlier, the definition of yoga is the union of the body and mind. The breath is the connection between the two. Calm and conscious breathing connects our physical state with our mental and emotional states.

A Lethargic Heart, Stagnant Circulation, and Disease

Glenda's yoga and guidelines for healthy eating have improved my life immensely.
I am a victim of multiple sclerosis and suffer from high cholesterol. After my diagnosis,
I went to a physiotherapist, but it did no good. I had very little stability and felt
depressed. The deterioration of my body and my mood continued, until I found Glenda.
Now, after two years of following Glenda's yoga routines, I've experienced improvements
in balance, flexibility, movement in my joints, and strength in my legs. Following
Glenda's nutritional guidelines has decreased my cholesterol from 250 to 175. I owe
so much to Glenda's knowledge of nutrition and yoga. My MS is stable—my mood
is changed.

— Courtney, 42

Heart attacks and strokes are the most common causes of death in Western society. The factors that contribute to heart disease and stroke—high cholesterol, arterial plaque, smoking, poor diet, inactivity, and stress—will all be addressed or eased by this yoga program.

By practicing this program, you will immediately boost your circulatory system, resulting in an increased heart rate and increased circulation. The program's nonstop movement is intensely aerobic, without being exhausting, because in yoga the heart is not stressed. Yoga is a naturally noninvasive aerobic workout. Throughout the workout, breathing is the key: Long, rhythmic breathing keeps your respiratory system functioning at optimum levels, dramatically improving circulation throughout the body.

But yoga does more than just get your heart pumping. Inverted exercises, such as the Shoulder Stand, reverse the flow of gravity, improve the blood supply to the lungs and the brain, and allow the legs and the heart to rest, for improved circulation. The pressure of the abdominal cavity against the diaphragm exercises the diaphragm and the heart muscles, as well.

INACTIVITY

After many years of not reaching my fitness goals, I became frustrated and for a period became very inactive. I felt fatigued, sluggish, and far beyond my years. I stumbled upon Glenda's class when a friend dragged me there. It was uphill all the way from there. I did what I could and built up slowly, but I started feeling the results pretty quickly, not just outwardly but inwardly, as well. This style of yoga has had a profound effect on me in every way. I am employed in the prison industry and have a tremendously stressful job. It has helped me stay focused throughout the day, and I am now better able to manage stressful situations.

— KATHRYN, 39

Here are three easy steps to looking and feeling young:

1. *Strengthen your muscles, using yoga's resistance training. (As the saying goes, "If you don't use it, you'll lose it.")*

2. *Lubricate your joints, through yoga's flexibility postures.*

3. *Work your tendons, through the full range of yoga movements.*

Joints and muscles not regularly put to work forget that they can work at all. Yoga reverses the deterioration of your muscles, joints, and tendons. The loss of even a small range of motion can have a serious impact on your life. People often have automobile accidents because they can't turn their bodies far enough to look behind them.

The majority of people with bad or injured backs have problems that result from weak back and stomach muscles. When you have a weak back, even simple, everyday chores can be very aging. But this condition can be easily prevented, or even cured, by stretching, toning, and moving—even if it's only for thirty minutes, three times each week.

INFLEXIBILITY

I have been an avid runner for over twenty years. I've run the New York marathon and several half-marathons. Six months ago, running forty or fifty miles a week, I started to feel like an old lady at 46. I noticed that my stride had gotten shorter and my hips were extremely tight. I started attending Glenda's classes two or three times a week. Since then I have noticed an unbelievable change, not only in my running, but in how I feel. I am no longer stiff when I stand. My flexibility continues to improve. My stride is much smoother, and I don't have the old stiffness in my hips. I have also noticed that my shoulders, arms, and stomach muscles are stronger. I feel so much better mentally and physically now that Glenda's yoga is in my life.

—NIKKI, 46

Running, cycling, golfing, and weight training without sufficient and proper stretching can be very aging. Your muscles are shortened and tightened, and your range of motion is restricted. Over time, this is an invitation to injury. By contrast, yoga takes you through the full range of motion of each part of your body, stretching and lengthening your muscles and moving every joint, resulting in flexibility.

It's critical to approach a stretching program with care, as stretching your muscles at random could cause injury and loss of, instead of increased, flexibility. In this program, we'll stretch when it's most beneficial: after exercise, when your body is warmed up.

GRAVITY

At 52, after many years of running and weight training, I felt fit, but was constantly battling pain and swollen, painful legs. I met Glenda, and she invited me to try her class. It was fun and demanding, as well as being one of the best things I've done for myself. I have never been in better shape and have none of the problems that used to

plague me, including varicose veins. I do four or five classes a week, and people con-
stantly ask me what I do to stay in such good shape. I enthusiastically tell them about
Glenda's class! In fact, my past trainer told me that yoga was certainly working, as he
had never seen me look so good.

My only complaint has been seeing myself in the rear mirror while doing Downward
Dog…frightening! Glenda solved that problem, too…she simply said, "Close your eyes."

—SUSAN, 52

Gravity is one of the strongest and most powerful forces on earth. The daily process of living on this planet promotes aging, as we experience a constant downward pull that ages our bodies. By reversing gravity through postures and muscle toning, we bring balance back to the body and reverse the disabling effects of the sagging organs and muscles—not to mention sagging faces, breasts, abdomens, and spines—that are the result of gravity's incessant pull.

This program also includes inverted postures, where your head is below your heart, that use gravity to restore equilibrium and pump richly oxygenated blood to your brain and upper body with less strain on your heart. We spend many hours each day with our bodies upright, and these inverted postures provide relief to those who suffer from varicose or enlarged veins, often caused by the heart's inability to maintain blood flow. Circulation is assisted by muscular activity when you exercise, while inactivity causes blood to accumulate in the legs. Yoga makes veins stretch and elongate, counteracting poor circulation.

EXCESSIVE WEIGHT

I have been an active participant in Glenda's yoga class for one and a half years, and
the results have been phenomenal. By modifying my nutritional intake and taking
Glenda's class three times a week, I have lost forty pounds and three dress sizes, and
I've completely reshaped my body. After years of weight lifting with a trainer, extreme
anaerobic conditioning drills, and hours upon hours of cardio, I now have the body

I have been striving for. I'm strong, toned, and flexible. I have more self-confidence, feel and look younger, have less stress, and have a higher energy level. I now can wear a size 10 off the rack, and that is such a great feeling. I love how I look, and I'm proud to say I did this because of Glenda's help. She truly made this journey very challenging, positive, and life enhancing.

—RANDI, 42

Being overweight makes people look old before their time. My program is the fastest calorie burner I've encountered in three decades of fitness training.

By combining yoga postures with nonstop movement, you not only work every muscle, you also sweat and breathe hard. This combination burns calories—fast. For maximum calorie burn, you really want to work out at least three days a week for thirty minutes each session. Once you begin that regimen and see the changes to your body and mind, you'll most likely be inspired to increase your workouts to four or five days each week.

Yoga stimulates and helps regulate every gland in the body by massaging and circulating freshly oxygenated blood to them. The glands that help regulate your weight are the thyroid gland (regulating your metabolic rate), the pancreas (controlling sugar and energy levels), and the pineal and pituitary glands (controlling appetite and moods). Properly stimulated through this program, the results will be quite profound, especially with regard to weight control.

Don't begin this program thinking about the number of pounds you want to lose. Just visualize getting a healthier body. The pounds will come off, and they'll stay off.

WHAT ELSE YOGA CAN DO

As if all of that isn't enough, there are still more age-defying benefits to consistent yoga practice.

Yoga for healthy and improved sex. Yoga poses stimulate and massage all the organs of the body, and as a result, yoga improves circulation to the male and female sexual organs. This results in greater sensitivity and performance.

A more flexible and strong body will also be able to react more favorably to its partner, obtain more freedom of movement, and be more conscious and confident with itself, at any age.

Stress is a major cause of sexual problems, decreasing your hunger for love-making. Yoga is an amazing stress reliever when practiced often. Enjoy the beautiful body you have been gifted with, and explore all its possibilities!

Yoga for avoiding the disabling effects of menopause. As a stress reliever, yoga has few equals, especially for women in or approaching menopause. Yoga balances the endocrine system and reduces the effects of menopausal hormonal changes. Coupled with a healthy, sugar-free diet, yoga can help you keep your blood-sugar levels constant, avoiding the high peaks and crashing lows that control your moods.

All the symptoms associated with menstruation and menopause can be reduced or alleviated by practicing yoga. Yoga poses are excellent for the reproductive organs, massaging and increasing blood to these areas. Forward bends, backbends, and stretches, especially those in which the hips are opened, are very beneficial. The seated and prone spinal twists improve the functioning of the adrenal glands and help increase estrogen in the body. Inverted postures such as the Shoulder Stand and Legs Against the Wall Pose have a beneficial effect on the glands of the endocrine system, massaging the thyroid and parathyroid, which regulate cell function. This also boosts the immune system.

Hot flashes and night sweats experienced by menopausal women are also greatly reduced by practicing the Shoulder Stand or Legs Against the Wall Pose. These poses are included at the end of Routine 3, to be done before Savasana (the relaxation period). Only those who do not have high blood pressure or associated symptoms should do the Shoulder Stand. During the yoga routine, and especially during each routine's closing Savasana, women need to give themselves quiet time and to be patient with and nurturing toward themselves.

HOW TO USE THIS BOOK

This program is designed to be used either alone or in conjunction with any other exercise routine. The book is divided into routines and chapters. Think of the book as a user-friendly companion that will support and guide you through the various poses. Each of the three routines includes a strength-building, cardiovascular, toning, sculpting, flexibility, and mind-body session. The routines are not divided up by what body part is being worked, but in combination, the poses in a full routine will work every part of the body for maximum effect.

Routine 1 is Beginner, Routine 2 is Intermediate, and Routine 3 is Advanced. The initial program for the first three weeks is designed to get you familiar with the poses and their sequence. In the first week, only practice Routine 1, ideally three times. (It should take you approximately 30 minutes per routine, no matter which routine you're practicing.) In the second week, practice only Routine 2, three times. In the third week, practice Routine 3, three times.

After you've completed the first cycle of routines, practice the routines in order each week (for example, Routine 1 on Monday, Routine 2 on Wednesday, and Routine 3 on Friday), for a total of three sessions each week. Each session should take you approximately 30 minutes. By doing all three routines each week, you will improve your body's ability to gain strength and flexibility. Take each routine step by step, and the results will be astounding.

Each routine will present you with different challenges. These are designed to take you to higher levels of achievement. And though each routine is equally challenging in its own way, taken together, these routines form the complete antiaging workout. Adding additional challenges is something you can do at your own discretion. You can always add more breaths or more repetitions when you feel ready.

At all times, listen to your body. It will tell you how fast to proceed. Every individual's body is different, and each person's level of fitness or lack of fitness is different. Enjoy the journey toward fitness. Even if you can only get through ten minutes a day, go at that pace until you can master more. You will progress.

Every minute that you move counts, just as every inch that you move deeper into the strengthening and flexibility poses counts.

Here are a few strategies to help maximize the results of this program:

- Establish a regular time for your sessions, at least three times a week, and stay consistent from week to week.

- Avoid eating before practicing. Wait about two hours after a heavy meal or one hour after a light one before you begin.

- Follow the instructions and get into the postures carefully, never forcing or flinging yourself into a posture. Practice using controlled movements.

- Breathe deeply through your nose and use unbroken rhythmic breathing throughout your practice. Be conscious of not holding your breath, as it tightens the body.

- Stand or sit tall in all the postures. Elongate your spine for correct alignment. The weight of your body should be distributed evenly. When you extend your spine, more space is created between the vertebrae, allowing greater freedom of movement.

- Truly follow the directions given for each pose. This information is crucial for the foundation of the pose, and it allows you to get the maximum benefit of the pose.

- Do not bounce in stretches. Bouncing will cause the muscles to shorten in a protection reflex, and overstretching can lead to an injury.

- Always lift, lengthen, and extend the body in each pose.

- Keep a chart of your progress. A visual record of how many times a week and for how long each day you are practicing will motivate you and help you keep track of what you've accomplished.

- For encouragement and support, refer to the captions of the photographs accompanying each pose. These will tell you why you are working that posture and exactly what inward and outward rewards you can expect to gain for your efforts.

- Listen to your body. Modify any poses as recommended if you feel stress. If your muscles are not strong enough to perform an exercise properly, your body will compensate by using other muscles, which could lead to injury. So take it slowly and modify as needed until you build more strength.

The program is simple and easy to follow, and your new youthful appearance and attitude will be your reward and your motivation to continue. Now, let's get started.

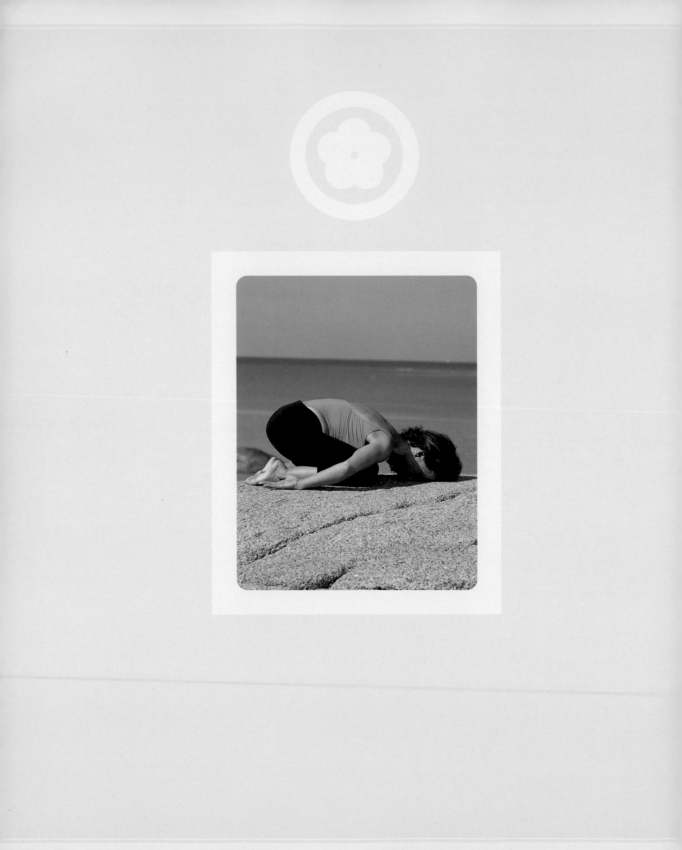

Chapter 3

Routine 1: Beginner

The very first step in any routine is to warm up the body. We accomplish this with Child's Pose and Cat's Pose, which stretch the spine and create suppleness. When these two poses are done before a routine, they release any stiffness in the back. We then proceed to the moves that will stretch your spine, shoulders, hips, and hamstring muscles effectively. It's very important to warm up and stretch, just for a few minutes, before attempting any of the routines described in this book.

After warming up the body and stretching, we will do some Sun Salutations, to start the cardiovascular effect with the movement of the body. Only then do we proceed to the different postures for each routine.

The Warrior Poses are incorporated only in Routine 1, so you can start building strength in your back, legs, hips, arms, and shoulders. Practicing these poses will start to improve your balance, to get you ready for Routine 2. Your stamina will start to ignite. In the Warrior Poses, we do counter poses—the Revolved Triangle and the Revolved Side Angle Pose—in which the spine is rotated. The poses strengthen and stretch the spine, preparing you for the backbends in Routine 3.

Before you get started, keep the following points in mind, as they will help you stay on track with your new, life-changing yoga program:

- During your three designated thirty-minute sessions each week, unplug the phone and lock the door. This is going to be a half-hour out of your day that is 100% "Me time."

- Expect peace and relaxation for those thirty minutes. Make your workout something to look forward to.

- Be committed to your schedule; consistency and structure are absolutely key.

- Buy one or two CDs of whatever kind of music inspires you. To get in the mood for your workout, start by playing the music that works for you. You'll also need a yoga mat, even if you work out on a carpeted floor.

- When you are very comfortable with the routine and you need more of a challenge, increase your workout time and intensity. Don't be intimidated by this thought when you're just beginning. Remember: You'll be hungry for the increase!

- Control the temperature of your workout room. The temperature should not go below 75° or over 78°F. Muscles respond most favorably to a warm environment, and heat causes the body to sweat. Sweat removes toxins and other impurities from the body. Body heat is an important component in making your muscles, tendons, and joints more pliable. The room you practice in should be warm, but not hot. Avoid drafty or overly air-conditioned rooms, as cold air on your muscles can be damaging and impair flexibility.

- Tell your spouse, boyfriend, girlfriend, children, or significant other what you're planning to accomplish. Tell them that you are accepting the challenge of being consistent with your workout, doing it three times a week for thirty-minute intervals. Discuss your challenges openly, and let your friends know that you may need a little push from time to time. You will only need their encouragement in the beginning stages because after that, your results will be your true motivator. This workout will become second nature to you.

If you've done yoga before, you've probably already heard the names of some of these poses. But for the uninitiated, we'll start each routine with a few definitions.

SUN SALUTATIONS. These are a series of poses synchronized with the breath in a flowing rhythm; they heat up the body and obtain a cardiovascular effect.

During Sun Salutations, the muscles and joints are loosened and the spine and body are taken through both forward and backward bends, to create balance. Through the Sun Salutations you will start to build strength, stamina, endurance, and flexibility.

WARRIOR POSES. Practicing the various Warrior Poses will build strength and endurance, alleviate stiffness in your neck and shoulders, and help improve flexibility in your knees, hip joints, and spine. This will result in an increased range of motion throughout your body. In Revolved Triangle Pose specifically, the internal organs are massaged and rejuvenated.

WARM-DOWN STRETCHING. These standing and seated poses are intense stretches for the backside of the body, and they include the Standing Forward Bend and Seated Head to Knee Poses. These lengthen and stretch the hamstrings, back muscles, and spine, and they're vital to include at the end of a routine.

SPINAL TWIST. Twisting is important to spinal health because it allows the intervertebral discs to move. As we get older, the water content between the discs decreases, and degenerative changes occurs in the discs. The yoga postures where we twist and stretch the spine allow the discs to suck in water and other nutrients. This prevents the discs from drying out, even into advanced age.

SAVASANA. Savasana allows you to totally relax and release any tension built up in your body by resting perfectly still and focusing your mind on internal sensations.

BREATHING

Breathing is an involuntarily act, we don't pay much attention to it. But breathing is the most vital activity of life. Most of us don't breathe efficiently, and as a result we only use a portion of our lung capacity.

When we're stressed, we take short, rapid, shallow breaths, and sometimes even hold our breath. Depriving our bodies of oxygen makes us feel run-down and fatigued. For optimal health, breathing should be deep, long, full, and rhythmic; it should completely fill and empty our lungs. Many of us need to relearn how to breathe properly, allowing our respiratory systems to function fully and completely. Breathing correctly relieves stress and anxiety and unleashes an enormous source of additional energy.

Here's a simple breathing exercise that's a great antidote to anxiety. Whenever you find yourself in a stressful situation, try this three-part breath:

1. *Inhale, filling your lungs completely with air, and hold the breath for a few seconds.*

2. *Exhale, slowly releasing the air from your lungs, emptying your lungs completely.*

3. *Repeat until you are out of the stressful situation.*

In yoga, there's a name for proper breathing. It's called pranayama, which is a Sanskrit term for "breath control." By controlling your breath, you can calm and relax your mind and body.

With the yoga poses, we use what is called a complete yoga breath. While practicing this breath, remember to keep your abdominal muscles firm and slightly contracted; they should be engaged throughout the breathing cycle. Breathe in an unbroken rhythm through your nose, keeping your mouth closed. During the routine, stay focused on not holding your breath.

1. *Inhale, expanding your chest and lifting your ribcage.*

2. *Exhale, feeling your chest sink and your lungs contract.*

One inhalation and one exhalation makes one breath. This yoga breath is what I'm referring to when I mention breath during the routines. The program is designed to coordinate the breath with the postures.

Now that we've covered the basics, you're ready to begin the first routine.

ROUTINE 1

Child's Pose

Child's Pose is a resting pose. It is essential at the beginning, middle, and end of a practice session. When your muscles are contracted, lactic acid is produced as a result of a decrease in oxygen to your muscles. This causes fatigue. As your muscles relax, however, oxygen is immediately brought to them and lactic acid is reduced. Relaxing and resting even for a short time in the middle of any form of exercise will change your workout by making you more energized and by allowing your muscles time to recover.

DIRECTIONS

1	Kneel on the floor and bring your buttocks toward your heels.
2	Place your arms lengthwise, alongside your body.
3	Stretch your chin forward and gently lower your forehead to the floor, rounding your spine and shoulders.
4	Relax your neck muscles and relax into the pose. Hold the pose for 3 breaths.

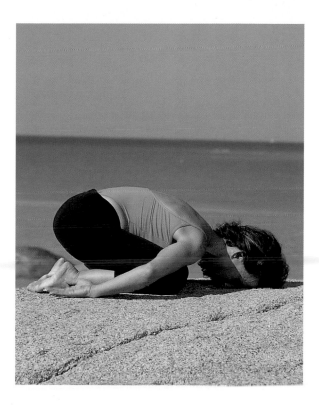

CHILD'S POSE stretches your back muscles, releases tension in your neck and shoulders, and increases flexibility of your hip joints. It also slows down your heart rate and calms emotions.

❋ MODIFICATION

If your forehead does not touch the floor when your buttocks are close to your heels, open your knees slightly, allowing your forehead to touch the floor. Place a pillow under your head, if necessary, until you gain the necessary flexibility.

ANTIAGING TIP

Child's Pose is a relaxing, tension-releasing pose. It's a good first step toward a youthful and relaxed body and mind.

Cat's Pose

This pose warms up the spine and starts to create a little movement there.

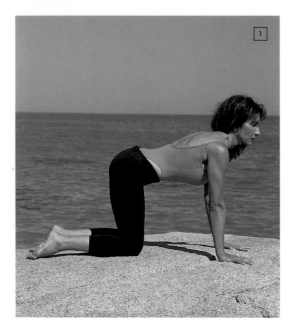

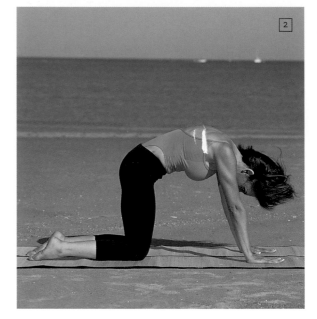

DIRECTIONS

1 Get on your hands and knees, with your palms under your shoulders and your knees under your hips.

2 Inhale, contract your abdominal muscles, and round your back, dropping your head toward the ground.

3 Exhale, release your abdominal muscles, arch your spine, and lift your head, sticking your buttocks out and up. All of the arching and rounding of your spine should initiate from your pelvis.

4 Repeat the pose 3 times.

From Cat's Pose, straighten your legs and raise your hips for the next pose, Downward Facing Dog.

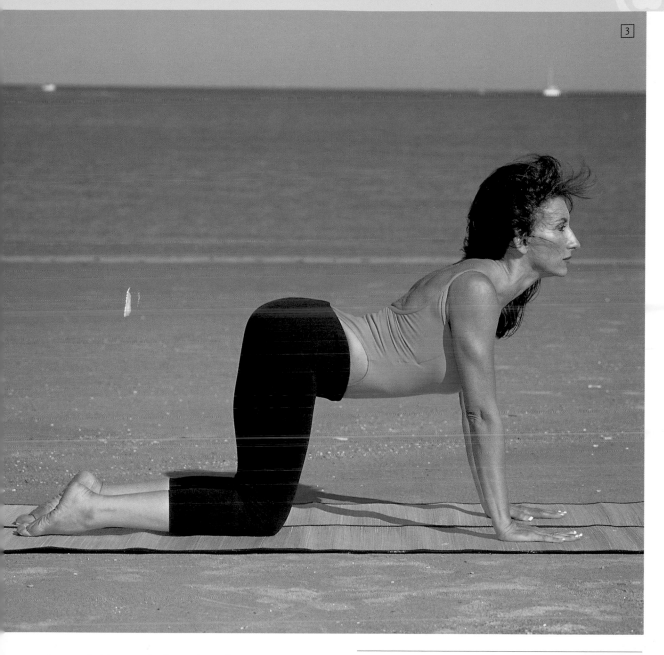

3

CAT'S POSE stretches your back muscles and prepares your spine for more aggressive poses.

Downward Facing Dog

This pose will lengthen your spine as it stretches your entire back. Even though it's usually used as a resting pose, it is a powerful pose that is necessary to fully stretch out your back between the other poses. Think of a dog stretching when he wakes up from a nap, stretching his hips way up in the air as he lengthens his body. It looks good, and it feels great.

DIRECTIONS

1 From Cat's Pose, straighten your legs and shift your weight toward your heels and hips. Reach your arms as far forward as you can, and keep your hands and feet shoulder-width apart.

2 Spread your fingers open, and make sure the palms of your hands are pressing evenly onto the floor.

3 Lift your tailbone upwards, keeping your knees bent as necessary.

4 Shift your weight backwards toward your hips, and pull your shoulder blades back toward your waist. Your weight should be evenly distributed between your hands and your feet.

5 Drop your head toward the floor and consciously release your neck muscles. Hold the pose for 5 breaths.

CHALLENGE

As time progresses, try and straighten your legs and bring your heels toward the floor

Move from Downward Facing Dog directly into the Forward Stretch.

DOWNWARD DOG POSE energizes and refreshes you in between postures. It strengthens the nerves and muscles in your upper body and legs, stretches the entire backside of your body, and increases blood supply to your head for clearer thinking.

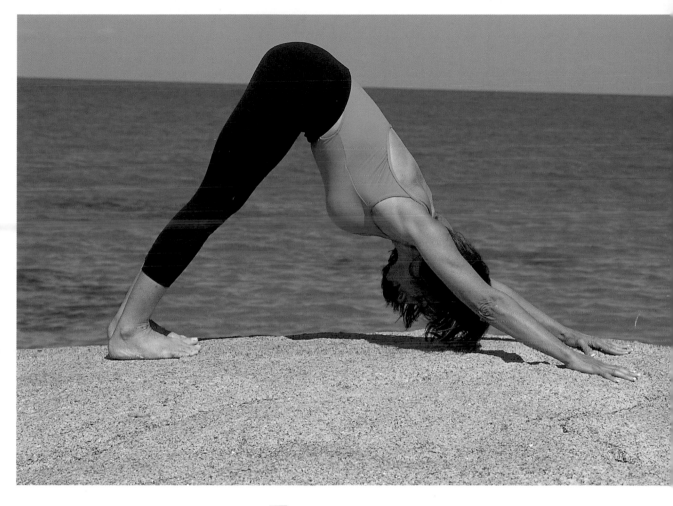

COMMON PROBLEMS

1. Not enough space between your hands and your legs.
2. Weight is not shifted backwards toward your hips and heels.
3. Hands aren't shoulder-width apart.
4. Feet aren't hip-width apart.

MODIFICATION

If you have wrist problems or carpal tunnel syndrome, buy a piece of spongy foam and cut a strip of it to the width of your yoga mat. Place this foam under the heels of your hands so that your wrists are slightly elevated. This will provide cushioning while shifting the weight away from your wrists and to the base of your palms. As you practice more, your wrists will get more flexible and the stiffness will ease, allowing you to stop using the foam support.

Three Warm-up Stretches:

Forward Stretch, Side Stretch, and Back Stretch

Always warm up with gentle stretching to prepare the body for more intense activity and reduce the risk of injury.

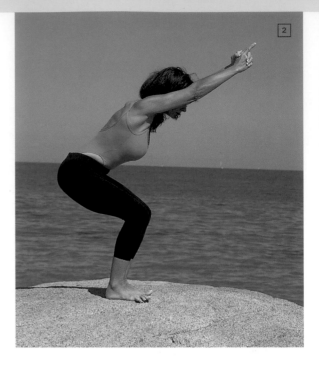

THE FORWARD STRETCH POSE releases tension and stretches your neck and shoulders.

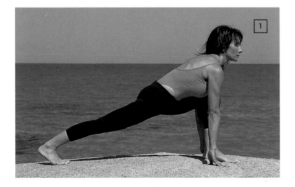

DIRECTIONS

1 Starting from Downward Facing Dog, raise your torso and bring your left foot in between your hands, then your right foot.

2 Keep your knees bent as you raise your torso and stretch your arms up and forward, for the Forward Stretch.

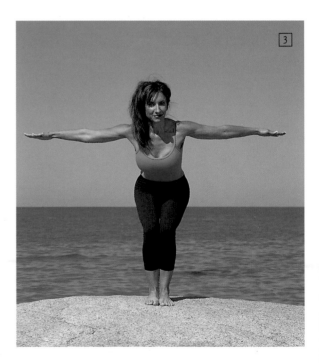

THE SIDE STRETCH POSE stretches your back and tones your stomach and torso muscles.

3 Holding your body in the same position, with knees still bent, stretch your arms all the way out to the side, for the Side Stretch.

4 Stretch your arms backwards toward your shoulders. Interlace your fingers and gently bend forward, straightening your legs as much as is comfortable, and releasing your head and neck muscles.

5 Stretch your arms a little higher away from your shoulders, for the Back Stretch. Hold for 3 breaths.

Slowly lift your torso to a standing position, still holding your hands and arms behind you, to prepare for the Lateral Side Stretch and Full Length Stretch.

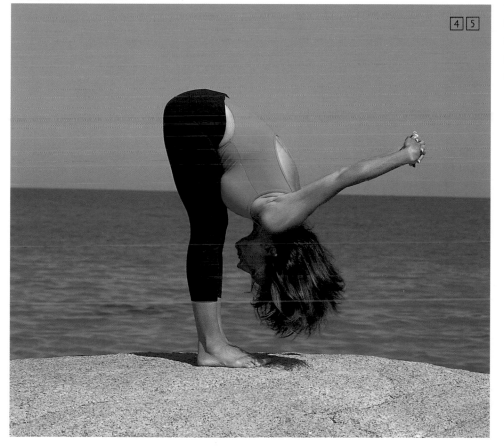

THE BACK STRETCH POSE 4 5 increases flexibility and releases tension and stiffness in your arms, neck, and shoulders.

Lateral Side Stretch and
Full Length Stretch

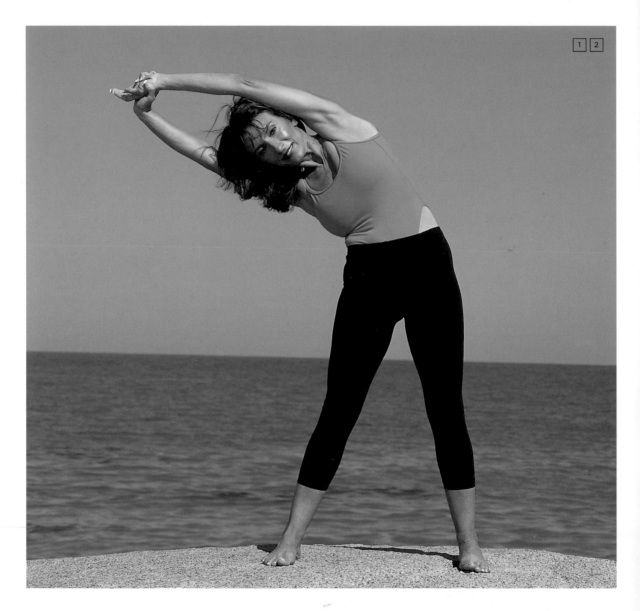

1 2

THE LATERAL SIDE AND FULL LENGTH STRETCHES increase flexibility to your spine, lengthen your torso, and loosen your leg and hip muscles.

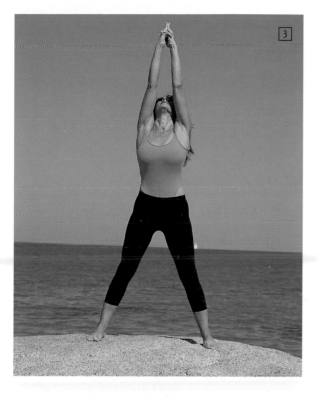

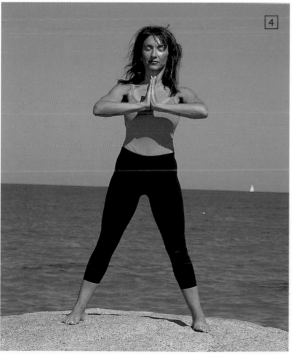

DIRECTIONS

1 Standing straight up, unclasp your hands and grab hold of your left wrist with your right hand. Stretch all the way over to the right.

2 Slowly return your body to standing straight, and switch hands, grabbing your right wrist with your left hand. Stretch all the way over to the left.

3 Slowly return your body to standing straight, release your hand, and interlace your fingers with your index fingers pointing upwards. Stretch your arms all the way over your head and gently release your head back. Feel the stretch from your waist all the way up to your pointed fingers.

4 Bring your hands to your heart center and close your eyes. Take 2 long, deep breaths, inhaling and exhaling completely, reaching down to the bottom part of your lungs.

Sun Salutation

Sun Salutations are made up of a series of poses, including standing poses, Plank, Chaturanga, Upward Facing Dog, and Downward Facing Dog. This series of poses awakens every inch of the body, imparting benefits to both the muscular and skeletal systems. Sun Salutations add suppleness to the spine, moving it in a backward and forward motion, and bring some flexibility to the shoulders, neck, arms, and hamstrings. They also jump-start the cardiovascular system through continuous movement of the body.

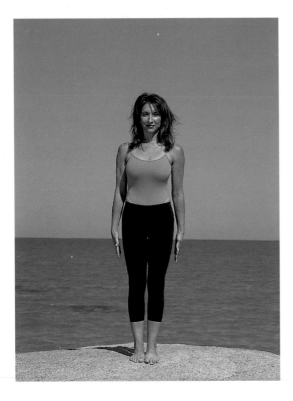 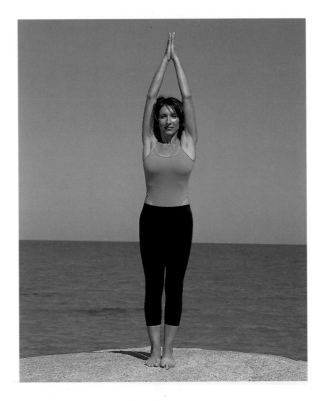

DIRECTIONS

1 Align your body, placing your feet together and your hands at your sides.

2 Inhale, roll your arms out with the palms facing out toward the ceiling, and bring your palms together overhead.

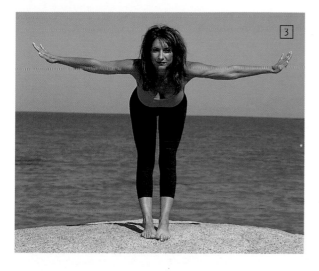

3 Exhale, roll your arms out to the side and toward the floor, and gently release your head down toward the floor, lengthening your spine. Place your hands flat on the floor beside your feet.

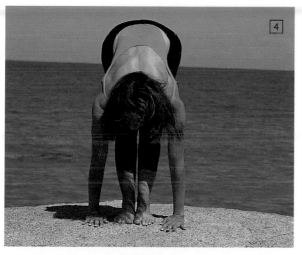

4 Inhale and lift your head up.

5 Exhale and release your head toward the floor.

Keep your hands on the floor and bring your right leg and then your left leg back, so your body is parallel to the floor and ready for Plank Pose.

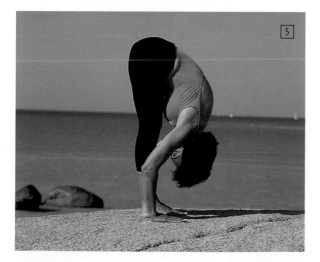

ANTIAGING TIP

A slow metabolism causes sluggishness and weight gain. Speeding up the body's metabolism is rejuvenating. These poses reverse the feeling of sluggishness from the inside out by stimulating your internal organs. That means that doing these poses will make you feel younger, slimmer, and more energized.

Plank Pose

(Sun Salutation, continued)

This is a weight-bearing pose. It will strengthen and prepare you for the other upper body poses that are more intense.

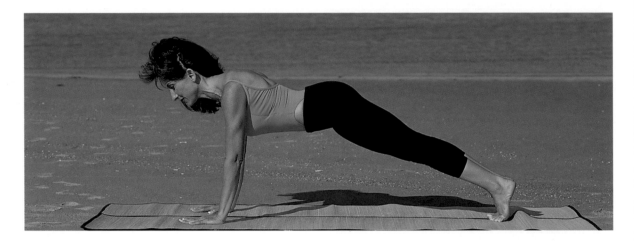

DIRECTIONS

1 Position your hands flat on the floor under your shoulders. Make sure they're pointing directly forward.

2 Tuck your toes under and come onto the balls of your feet, stretching through your heels.

3 Activate both thighs while keeping the back of your body really firm and flat.

4 Press firmly into your hands, and look toward the floor.

THE PLANK POSITION POSE increases upper body strength, develops upper back muscles, and is an excellent weight-bearing exercise for increasing bone mass.

ANTIAGING TIP

Because you support your body with just your hands and feet, this pose is tremendously strengthening for the wrists and toes, and it increases flexibility, too.

Continue directly into either the Modified Chaturanga or Challenge Chaturanga Pose.

Modified Chaturanga Pose

(Sun Salutation, continued)

Chaturanga is the Sanskrit term for a modified push-up. The pose will help you develop strength in your upper body and start to reshape your arms and shoulders.

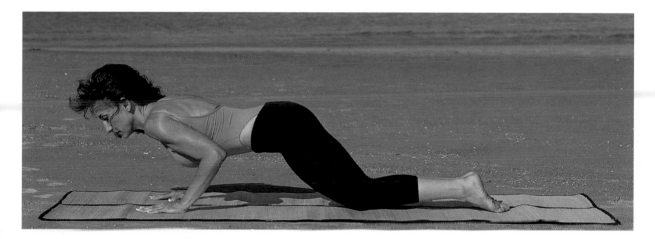

DIRECTIONS

1 Lower your knees to the floor, still keeping the muscles of your legs engaged.

2 Bend your elbows back, keeping them close to your body. Keep your shoulders square and gaze toward the floor.

3 Bend your elbows and bring your chest toward the floor, keeping your shoulders in line with your elbows, not lower, and keeping your body as straight as can be. Hold for 5 breaths.

THE MODIFIED CHATURANGA POSE builds upper body strength—it specifically strengthens your arms and wrists, and increases and improves bone density.

ANTIAGING TIP

This weight-bearing exercise will be a great asset to you in your battle to prevent or put a hold on osteoporosis.

Challenge Chaturanga Pose

(Sun Salutation, continued)

When you have sufficient strength, perform this pose in place of the Modified Chaturanga. This pose is used often, and needs special attention if you're going to master it.

DIRECTIONS

1 Remain in Plank Pose, with your knees off the floor.

2 Lower your upper body by bending your elbows, tucking them in, and hugging your ribcage. Continue to keep your body firm and supported; don't let it sag to the floor. If this happens, place your knees to the floor in Modified Chaturanga Pose.

3 Keep your elbows as close to your body as you can and your palms flat on the floor.

4 Lengthen your spine and keep your thighs active as you tighten your tummy muscles and gaze toward the floor. Hold the pose for 5 breaths.

COMMON PROBLEMS

1. Hands aren't directly under your shoulders.
2. Elbows aren't tucked in.
3. Not enough strength for Challenge Chaturanga.
4. Looking up, rather than gazing toward the floor.
5. Leading with your nose, rather than your chest, as you lower yourself toward the floor.
6. Allowing your shoulder blades to "cave in" toward each other.

From the Modified or Challenge Chaturanga, continue directly into Upward Facing Dog.

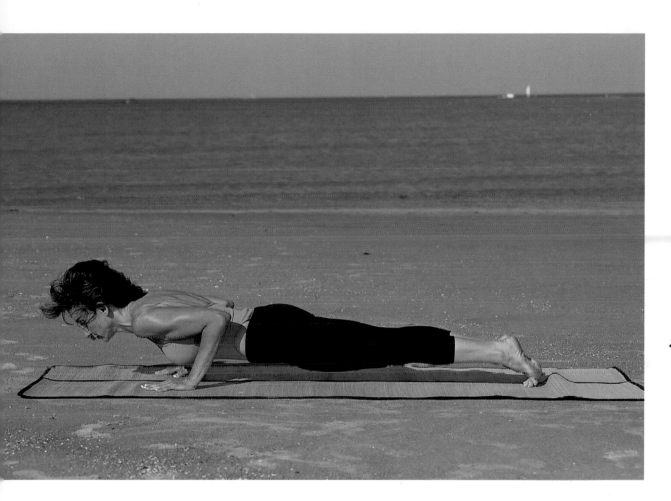

THE CHALLENGE CHATURANGA POSE, or yoga push-up,
builds strength in your arms and upper body and increases
mobility in the wrists.

Upward Facing Dog
Sun Salutation, continued

This pose really starts to warm up the spine with a gentle backbend. It will also open your chest and strengthen your arms and shoulders.

DIRECTIONS

1 From either Chaturanga Pose, scoop your chest and move your whole body forward and upward, rolling forward over the tops of your toes into Upward Facing Dog.

2 Open and lift your chest, straighten your arms, and lift your body so that only your hands and the tops of your feet support your body. Try and lift your thighs off the floor by tightening your thighs and buttocks.

3 Arch your spine and gaze directly in front of you, or gently drop your head back.

4 Curl your toes under, lift your hips, and stretch back into Downward Facing Dog.

5 Repeat the Sun Salutation series 2 or 3 times, remaining in the final position when you complete your repititions

MODIFICATION

If you cannot lift your thighs off the floor during Upward Facing Dog, begin by performing this pose with your thighs and the tops of your feet on the floor.

COMMON PROBLEMS

1. Hunching and rounding your shoulders so they're up around your ears.
2. Sinking the weight of your body into the floor.

Move Directly from Downward Facing Dog to Warrior Pose.

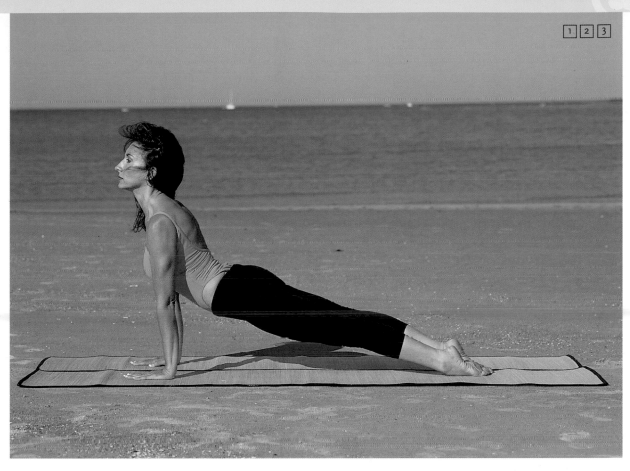

1 2 3

THE UPWARD FACING DOG POSE brings flexibility to your spine and blood to your pelvic region.

ANTIAGING TIP

The pose helps prevent arthritis of the spine by increasing flexibility and movement. This increased flexibility, along with an influx of blood to the pelvic region, will make you look and feel younger.

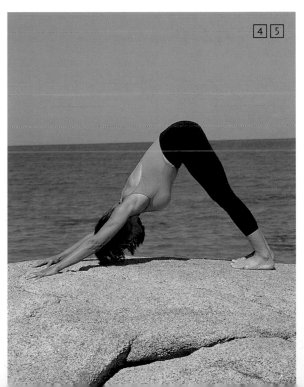

4 5

Warrior I

To keep the energy moving and create internal heat, try to maintain the fluidity of constant movement, flowing from one pose to another. Your ability to do this will increase as you become more familiar with the routine.

The next six poses are variations of the Warrior Poses. Warrior I builds strength in your entire body, especially your legs. The pose is called Warrior because it resembles a powerful warrior hero from a Hindu legend.

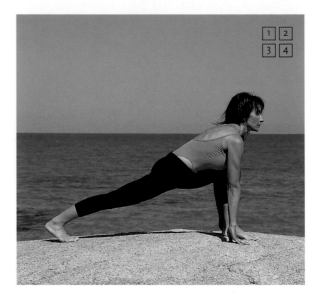

THE WARRIOR ONE POSE tones your thighs, awakens your spine, and opens your groin muscles. It also strengthens your knees and makes your ankles more flexible.

DIRECTIONS

1 From Downward Facing Dog, bring your left foot in between your hands. (Before you gain strength and balance, you may find you have to stand up first and then position yourself.)

2 Leave your right foot flat on the floor, but turn it out at a 45-degree angle.

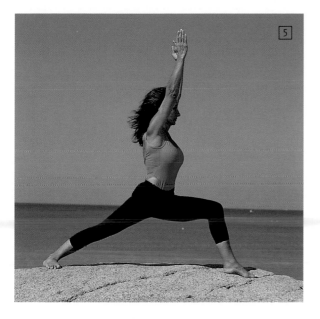

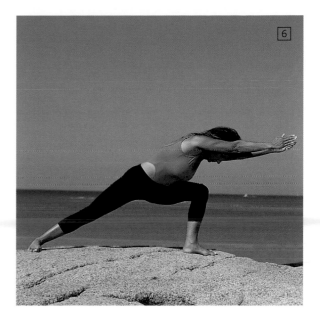

 Check the positioning of your feet—
they should be about 3 feet apart, and
should be directly under your fingertips when your arms are spread open.

4 Square your hips forward, point your
front foot directly ahead, and make
sure both your heels are in line with
each other.

5 Lift your arms above your head,
palms facing each other, hands shoulder-width apart. Bend your left knee
so it is directly above your ankle,
forming a 90-degree angle.

6 Bend forward from the waist, gazing
toward the ground.

7 Repeat Steps 5 and 6, reaching your
arms up again, and then bending forward from your waist with your arms
forward.

8 Bring your hands flat on each side
of your left foot, and bring your leg
back behind you into Plank Pose.

*From Plank Pose, perform one modified Sun
Salutation.*

Modified Sun Salutation

This is an abbreviated version of the Sun Salutation, eliminating the standing positions.

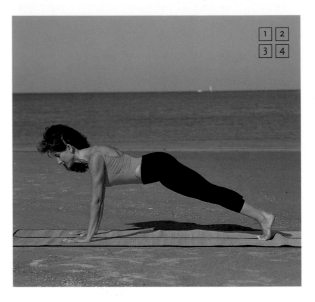

DIRECTIONS

1 In Plank Pose, position your hands on the floor directly under your shoulders. Make sure they're pointing directly forward.

2 Tuck your toes under and come onto the balls of your feet, stretching through your heels.

3 Activate both thighs while keeping the back of your body really firm and flat.

4 Press firmly into your hands, looking toward the floor.

5 Place your knees on the floor, still keeping the muscles of your legs engaged. (Alternatively, you can perform the Challenge Chaturanga Pose here if you are able.)

6 Bend your elbows back, keeping them close to your body. Keep your shoulders square and gaze toward the floor.

7 Bend your elbows and bring your chest toward the floor, keeping your shoulders in line with your elbows, not lower, and keeping your body as straight as can be. Hold for 5 breaths.

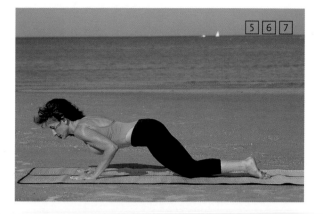

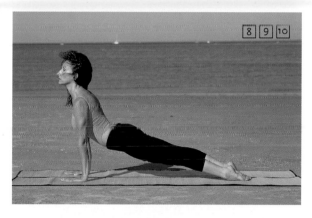

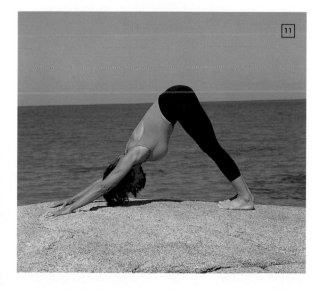

8 Scoop your chest and move your whole body forward and upward, rolling forward over the tops of your toes into Upward Facing Dog.

9 Open and lift your chest, straighten your arms, and lift your body so that only your hands and the tops of your feet support your body. Try and lift your thighs off the floor by tightening your thighs and buttocks.

10 Arch your spine and gaze directly in front of you, or gently drop your head back.

11 Curl your toes under, lift your hips, and stretch back into Downward Facing Dog.

From Downward Facing Dog, move directly into Warrior II.

Warrior II

DIRECTIONS

1 From Downward Facing Dog, bring your left foot in between your hands. (Before you gain strength and balance, you may find you have to stand up first and then position yourself.)

2 Leave your right foot flat on the floor.

3 Check the positioning of your feet—they should be about 3 feet apart, and should be directly under your fingertips when your arms are spread open.

4 Square your hips forward.

5 Bring your arms up to shoulder height, palms facing the floor, and rotate your torso so your arms are in line with your body and your legs.

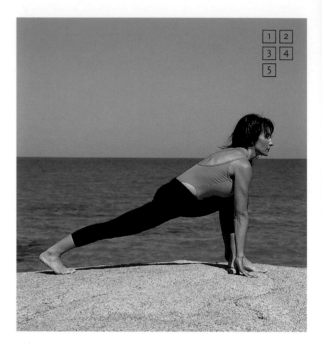

6 Bend your left knee so it is directly above your ankle, forming a 90-degree angle, and lower yourself into a lunge position. You may have to readjust your position, spreading feet wider apart, to achieve this alignment. Keep hips aligned.

7 Turn your head to the left, looking past your left hand. Hold the pose for 5 breaths.

Hold the final position as you transition into Reverse Warrior Pose.

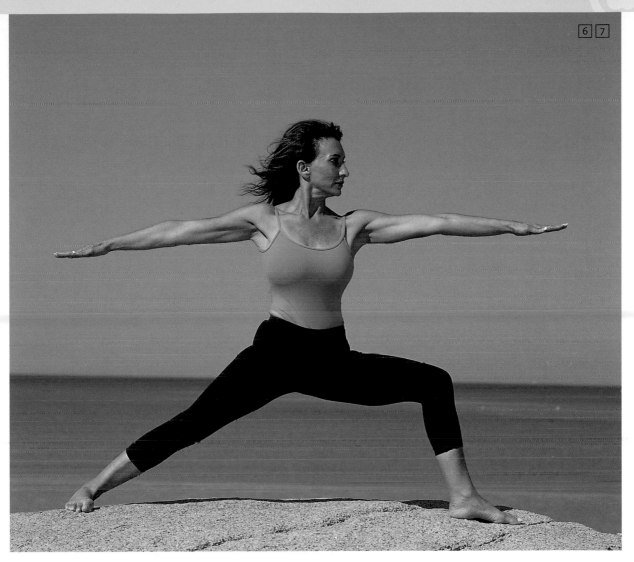

THE WARRIOR II POSE helps you develop stamina, strengthens your back and legs, and gives you an intense groin stretch.

ANTIAGING TIP

All the Warrior Poses are rejuvenating. By putting your hips and knees through their full range of movement, the poses help to distribute synovial fluid, lubricating the joints and removing stiffness.

COMMON PROBLEMS WITH ALL WARRIOR POSES

1. Hips aren't properly aligned.
2. Lunge isn't deep enough and the knee isn't in line with the ankle. The lunge should form a 90-degree angle, to get the full benefit of the pose.
3. Back knee is bent.
4. Front knee turns in.

Reverse Warrior Pose

This Warrior Pose includes a gentle backbend, to increase flexibility in your spine while building strength in your body.

DIRECTIONS

 1 From Warrior II, inhale and raise your left arm toward the ceiling, sliding your right arm alongside your right leg and gently bending back at the waist.

2 Exhale, and look up and back.

3 Let your lower body sink into the pose as your upper body lifts up toward the sky. Hold the pose for 5 breaths.

4 Return to Warrior II, with your arms at shoulder height and palms facing the floor; do not move the lower body and legs. Hold the pose for 5 breaths.

Stay in Warrior II to begin the Standing Lateral Pose.

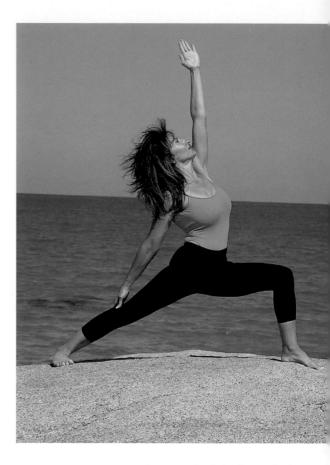

THE REVERSE WARRIOR POSE increases circulation in your back, brings flexibility and suppleness to your spine, strengthens your legs, and helps you develop balance.

ANTIAGING TIP

This is a great all-purpose pose. The stance builds tremendous strength while toning and shaping your legs, giving you a youthful body, and the backward bend gives you a more supple spine—so rejuvenating!

Standing Lateral Pose

This variation of Warrior creates a diagonal stretch in the upper body that helps build even more strength in the legs and thighs as you hold the pose.

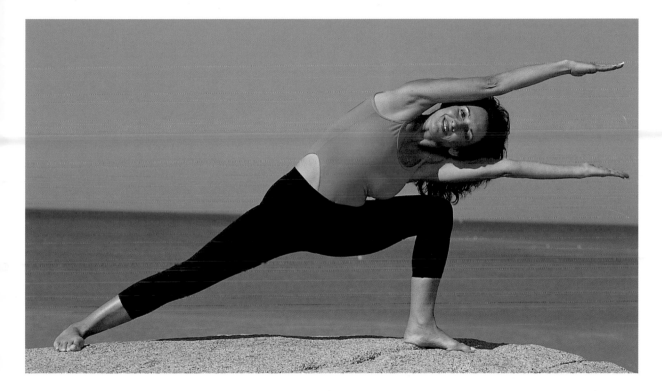

DIRECTIONS

1 From Warrior II, turn your left palm up to face the ceiling.

2 Inhale, and bend from the waist to your right side.

3 Bring your right arm all the way over, so it's parallel to your left arm and parallel to the floor. Exhale and hold the posture for 5 breaths.

4 Return your torso to an upright position and place your arms back at shoulder level, palms down, in Warrior II.

Extended Side Angle Pose

This dynamic diagonal stretch works the upper body while you strengthen and reshape your legs and thighs by holding the Warrior Pose.

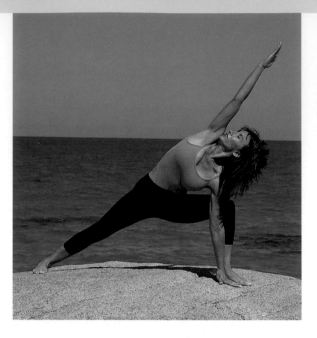

THE EXTENDED SIDE ANGLE POSE provides an intense stretch to your sides of the body and to your legs, opens your hips, and stretches your groin.

DIRECTIONS

1 From Warrior II, inhale, lean to your left, and place your left elbow in front of your left knee. Place your left hand flat on the floor next to the inside of your left foot.

2 Lift your right arm straight over your head, forming a straight line from your back heel all the way to your fingertips.

3 Exhale and turn your head up, looking under your right arm and toward the ceiling. Hold the pose for 5 breaths.

MODIFICATION

If looking up toward the ceiling bothers your neck, you can look down or in front of you.

ANTIAGING TIP

The Extended Side Angle Pose and the Revolved Side Angle Pose (below) are the most effective poses to increase the flexibility of the hip joint and the muscles of the side of the torso. These poses specifically target the last five vertebrae, stretching and strengthening them to help counteract lower back pain and lumbago rheumatism, both of which are aging conditions.

From this position, go directly into the Revolved Side Angle Pose.

Revolved Side Angle Pose

This is a dynamic, powerful stretch for your back muscles as you revolve or twist to the other side.

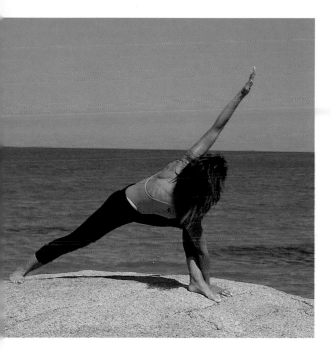

THE REVOLVED SIDE ANGLE POSE helps relieve lower back discomfort and increases flexibility in your hips.

DIRECTIONS

1 From Extended Side Angle Pose, inhale and twist your torso from the waist, bringing your right hand on the outside of your left foot.

2 With your knee still bent at a 90-degree angle, exhale and bring your left arm straight up and a little over to a 45-degree angle. This will give you an extended side stretch. Hold the pose for 5 breaths. You will feel your spine moving and becoming supple.

 MODIFICATION

If you cannot twist the body so that your hand is on the outside of your foot, twist and bring your hand to the inside of your foot.

Hold this position and move into Standing Head to Knee Pose.

Standing Head to Knee Pose

This pose is actually a forward bend, and it really stretches out those hamstrings.

DIRECTIONS

1 From Revolved Side Angle Pose, bring the torso up and straighten both legs, keeping your thighs active, front toe still facing forward and back foot still flat and at a 45-degree angle.

2 Square your hips and shoulders forward, straighten your arms behind your back, and interlace your hands with your palms facing in.

3 Inhale, and lengthen through your entire spine, from your tailbone to your head.

4 Exhale, and bend your body forward from your hips. Lift your tailbone up toward the ceiling, leading with your chest toward your leg, and surrender your head toward the floor. Draw your arms over your head as high as possible.

5 Keep your elbows straight as you lift your arms, and keep your head and spine in a straight line. Release your neck muscles, keeping them soft. Hold the pose for 5 breaths.

 MODIFICATION

If you cannot perform the pose with your hands interlaced behind your back, begin with your hands on your waist.

COMMON PROBLEMS

1. Leading with your head and not your chest.
2. Not lengthening your spine as you fold forward.

From Standing Head to Knee Pose, bend your front knee and come onto the floor into Child's Pose.

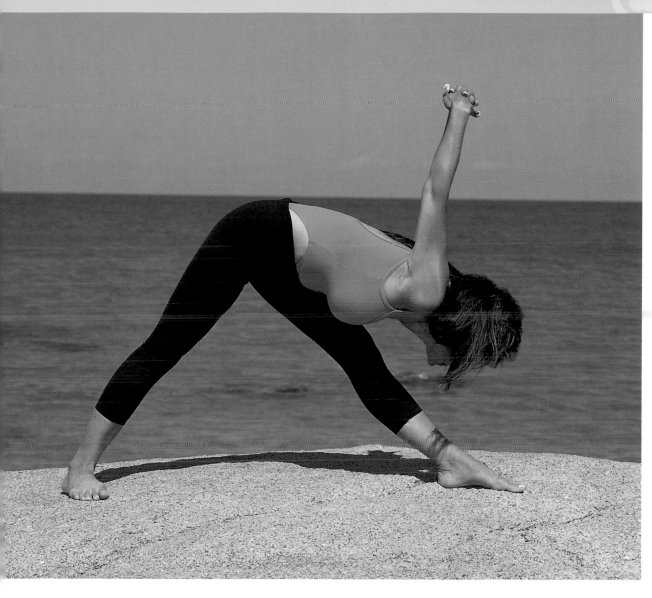

ANTIAGING TIP

Sciatica can be cured and prevented with poses such as this one, which stretches and strengthens the sciatic nerves and tendons of the leg.

THE STANDING HEAD TO KNEE POSE lengthens your legs, hips, and the whole backside of your body. This pose gives your hamstrings a particularly intense stretch.

Child's Pose

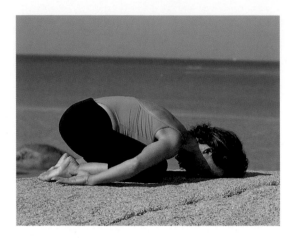

DIRECTIONS

1 Kneel on the floor and bring your buttocks toward your heels.

2 Place your arms lengthwise, alongside to your body.

3 Stretch your chin forward and gently lower your forehead to the floor, rounding your spine and shoulders.

4 Relax your neck muscles and relax into the pose. Hold the pose for 3 breaths.

Repeat the series, from Warrior I through Child's Pose, with your right leg before continuing on with the rest of Routine 1.

Triangle Pose

As the name implies, in this pose you form an extended triangle with your body. It is a challenging posture that incorporates a forward bend, balance, and stretching.

DIRECTIONS

1 Place your feet about 3 feet apart. Keep both legs straight and extend your arms straight out from your shoulders, palms facing toward the floor and quadriceps actively contracted.

2 Inhale, and shift your torso to the left, placing your left hand flat on the floor on the outside of your left foot.

3 Reach your right arm up toward the ceiling, extending your spine. Open your chest and look up toward your arm. Lengthen your head away from your tailbone, making your torso as parallel to the floor as possible.

4 Exhale, and open up your chest as far as you can toward the ceiling. The weight of your body should be toward the back of your back heel. Hold the pose for 5 breaths.

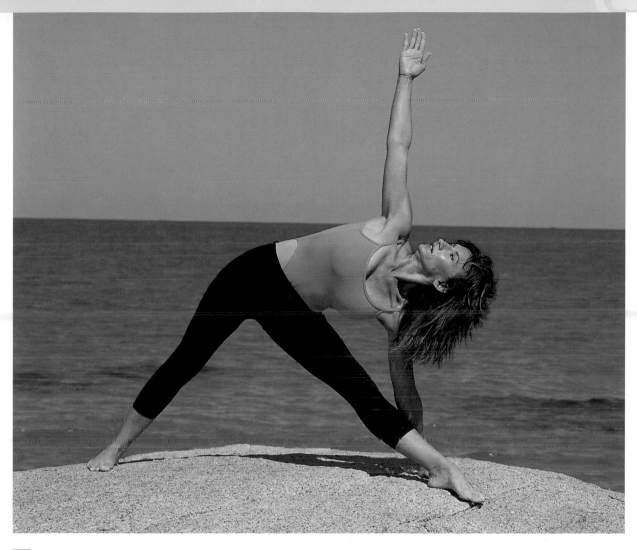

✤ MODIFICATIONS

If you can't reach the floor with a flat hand, either place a block under your hand or hold onto your ankle or shin. If it hurts your neck to look up toward your extended arm, look forward or toward the floor.

COMMON PROBLEMS

1. Bad posture, including rounding of the back.
2. Not extending the spine from the head through to the tailbone.
3. Letting your torso face the floor instead of facing sideways.

THE TRIANGLE POSE strengthens your feet, ankles, and knees, opens your hips and chest, and elongates your spine.

ANTIAGING TIP

As we age, our hips and chest close and become tight. This pose reverses that trend by opening and stretching the whole body.

From this position, move directly into Revolved Triangle Pose.

Revolved Triangle Pose

This is a forward bend, a balancing pose, and a twist. It's the counter pose for the triangle posture.

DIRECTIONS

1 While still in Triangle Pose, inhale and twist your torso, rotating your right arm all the way over to the outside of your left foot.

2 Pull your right hip back as you look up and over your left shoulder.

3 Exhale as you stretch your arms and shoulders away from your breastbone, extending your left arm toward the ceiling. Hold the pose for 5 breaths.

✿ MODIFICATION

If you cannot reach the floor, reach for your leg, shin, or foot, or use a yoga block or a shoebox to rest your hand on.

COMMON PROBLEMS

1. Rounding the spine, instead of lengthening from the tailbone through to the top of your head.
2. Not bending from your hips.
3. Twisting from the shoulders, rather than the hips and torso.

Repeat the Triangle and Revolved Triangle Poses with your right leg, moving from your final position into Standing Forward Bend Pose.

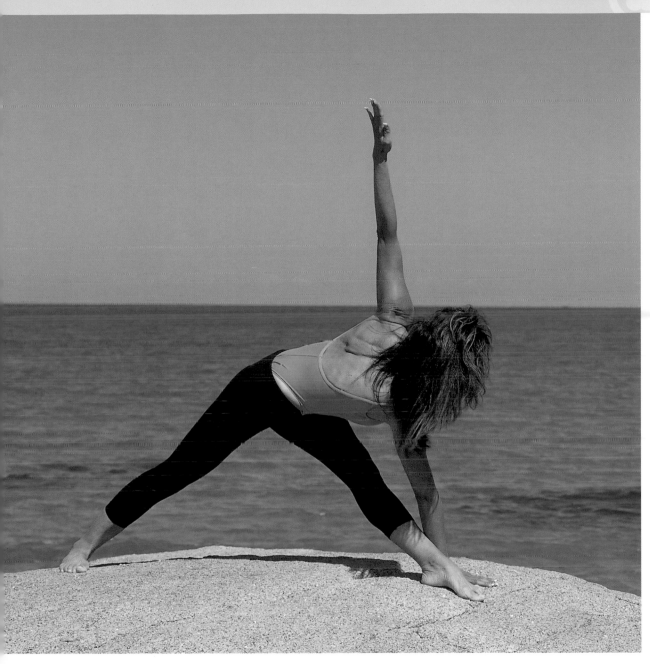

THE REVOLVED TRIANGLE POSE tones your waistline, helps to relieve lower back pain, increases flexibility in your hips, strengthens your pelvic are and massages your reproductive organs.

ANTIAGING TIP

This pose helps prevent and relieve lower back discomfort by increasing flexibility in the hips and legs.

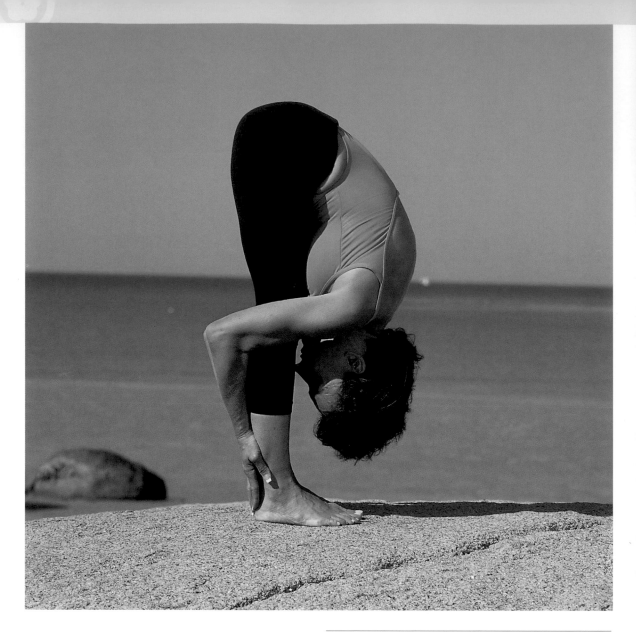

THE STANDING FORWARD BEND strengthens your spine and legs and loosens your hamstrings, massages your pelvic organs, stretches and strengthens your spine, and increases blood flow to your head for clearer thinking.

ANTIAGING TIP

As your hamstrings and back muscles lengthen, strengthen, and stretch, your spine will be rejuvenated and you'll feel increased flexibility throughout your body.

Standing Forward Bend Pose

This is an inverted posture, so you fold forward and as a result get an intense stretch to your hamstring muscles. This will also lengthen, strengthen, and stretch your back, opening every vertebra in your spine.

DIRECTIONS

1 From Revolved Triangle Pose with your right foot forward, bend your right knee and bring both hands to either side of your foot. Bring your left foot forward and straighten your legs.

2 Bring your arms out to the side and your hands to your heart center, standing upright.

3 Inhale and lift your arms over your head.

4 Exhale and fold forward from the hips (not from the middle of the back), keeping your spine straight. Relax your hip joints so your body bends without your back curving, and place your hands on the floor next to your feet, or hold your shins or ankles.

5 Lift your buttocks and lower your head to your shins. Relax your abdominal muscles and ease into the pose without forcing it. Hold the pose for 5 breaths.

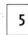 **MODIFICATION**

Initially, bend your legs enough to release any tension in your back. Work toward having your legs completely straight in the final posture.

COMMON PROBLEMS

1. Back is rounded.
2. Weight of your body is on your heels.
3. Head is forced toward your knees.
4. Hips are not supported and are dropping back.
5. Feet are apart.

Lying Down Hip Stretch

This is a great hip opener. It may seem like a simple pose, but it's very powerful.

DIRECTIONS

1 Lie flat on your back with the sole of your right foot flat on the floor.

2 Place your left ankle on top of your right knee, and flex your left foot.

3 Interlace your fingers around the top of your right knee, drawing your knee toward your chest. The closer you bring your knee in toward your chest, the greater the stretch to your hips. Hold the pose for 10 breaths.

4 Repeat with the opposite leg.

ANTIAGING TIP

This stretch will give you overall agility and freedom of movement, and nothing will make you feel younger than that!

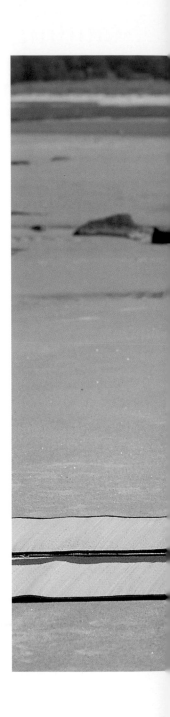

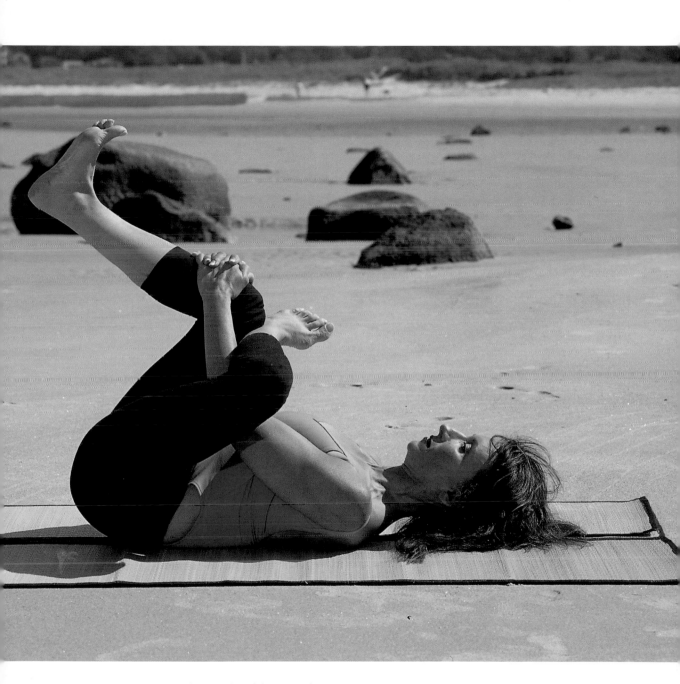

THE LYING DOWN HIP STRETCH stretches your hip abductors and rotator
muscles of the buttocks, and opens your hips, which releases lower
back tension.

Seated Head to Knee Pose

As the name suggests, you bring your head toward your knees, or your chest toward your thighs, for gaining flexibility of the spine and stretching out those hamstrings.

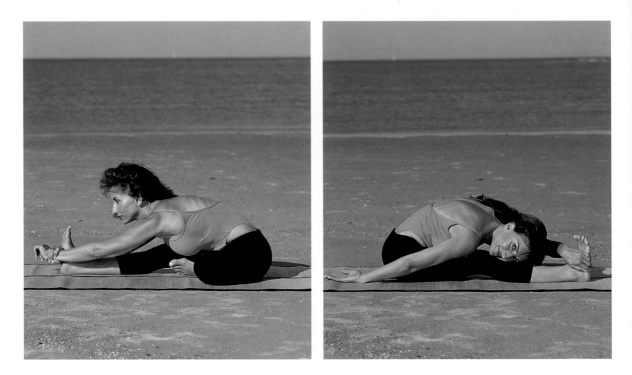

THE SEATED HEAD TO KNEE POSE increases flexibility to lower back and hamstrings, strengthens and elongates your spine, improves flexibility of your knees and hip joints, and improves digestion and circulation of bowels.

ANTIAGING TIP

If you're very stiff or your hamstrings are very tight, you'll initially find this pose very challenging. But inch by inch you'll get more flexible, and that newfound flexibility will prevent long-term injury and premature aging.

DIRECTIONS

1 Sit with your legs outstretched and feet together, pressing down evenly on the floor with your buttock bones.

2 Bend your left leg, and place the sole of your left foot against the inside of your right thigh. Keep your right knee on the floor as much as possible.

3 Inhale and raise both arms overhead as you lift and lengthen your spine forward.

4 Exhale, and bend forward from your hips, followed by your lower back, your middle back, and your upper back. Rest your chest as close to your knee as you can.

5 Hold the toes of your extended foot, and gradually ease further forward, clasping your hands around the sole of the foot. Hold the pose for 5 breaths.

6 Now place your left hand on the outside of your right foot or ankle, wherever you can reach. Place your right hand on the floor behind you and twist your body over, lifting and stretching out to the side. Your ultimate goal is for your left ear to meet your right knee. Hold the pose for 5 breaths.

7 Repeat with the opposite leg.

MODIFICATION
Loop a small towel around the foot of your extended leg. Hold the towel ends with both hands while sitting upright, then ease yourself forward.

CHALLENGE
Hold the pose for 10 breaths.

COMMON PROBLEM
Hunching your back. Do not to bend all the way to reach your ankle if you cannot maintain the correct posture.

Spinal Twist

In this posture, you will stretch your back from top to bottom, and as you twist and turn you will nourish your spinal discs.

The most important element of any twisting pose is that the spine be lengthened as it turns. Imagine the form of a spiral staircase as you perform these poses, and you will create space between your vertebrae. Maintain good posture and never force a twisting pose. Also, never lead a twist with your head, but allow your head to follow the twist; this will prevent neck strain.

DIRECTIONS

1 Sit tall and straight, with your spine as straight as can be and both legs extended forward.

2 Bend your left leg and drop your knee to the floor.

3 Wrap your right leg around, so your right ankle is on the outside of your left knee and your right foot is flat on the floor.

4 Place your left elbow on the outside of your right knee, drawing your right knee toward your chest and releasing your right hip toward the floor.

5 Lean back on your right hand, arm straight and close to your body.

6 Inhale, and extend and lengthen your spine.

7 Exhale, and rotate your body further to the right, looking over your right shoulder. Hold the pose for 5 breaths, twisting a little further with each exhalation.

8 Repeat on the other side, bending your right leg under and wrapping your left leg around it.

 MODIFICATION

In Step 2, instead of bending your left leg, leave it straight, and then wrap your right leg over it.

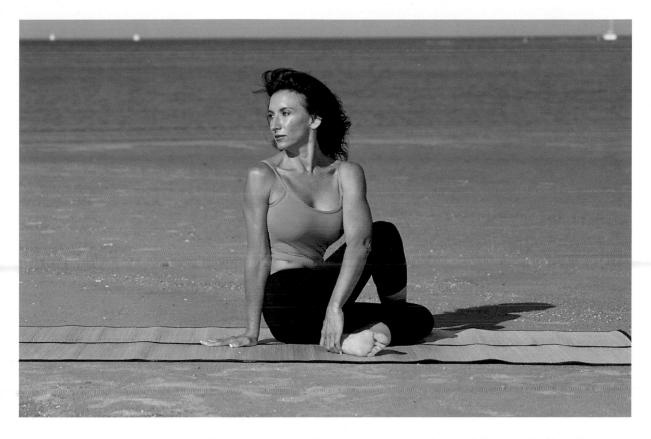

THE SPINAL TWIST exercises the entire back from top to bottom, helping to keep your spine elastic and alleviating shoulder stiffness. It also stimulates internal organs, improves digestion, and tones your stomach muscles.

COMMON PROBLEMS

1. Bad posture; make sure your spine is straight.

2. Leaning your body backward, rather than sitting straight in your twist.

3. Looking ahead instead of turning your head in the direction of the twist.

4. Allowing your head to droop, rather than holding it erect.

5. Rounding and hunching your shoulders, rather than keeping them down and away from your ears and parallel to the floor.

ANTIAGING TIP

This simple twist is invaluable for

weak and painful backs.

Savasana, or Corpse Pose

This is an important pose to end your session with because it is a stress reliever and because it lets all the body systems, including circulation and breathing, go back to normal.

Deep relaxation is an incredible stress reliever because it quiets the mind and leads to slower, fuller breathing; slower heartbeat; a quieted nervous system; and a calmer mind. As you progress, there will be more and more space between all that noisy chatter in your mind and your thoughts.

DIRECTIONS

1 Lie flat on your back with your feet apart and your toes relaxed and facing out.

2 Place your arms slightly out from your sides, with your palms up.

3 Close your eyes and consciously release and relax each and every muscle, transferring all the weight of your body to the floor.

4 Slowly bring your focus to your breath, and feel the rhythmic movement of your body as you breathe in and out. Really get in touch with your body and your breath, holding the pose for 5 to 10 minutes.

5 Wrap your arms around your knees, drawing them into your chest, and roll to your right side into a fetal position.

From this position, roll onto your knees to prepare for Child's Pose.

MODIFICATION

If your lower back feels uncomfortable lying in Savasana, bend your knees instead of straightening your legs.

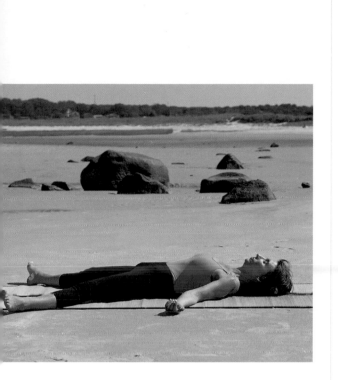

THE SAVASANA POSE instills the process of releasing and letting go, and helps you develop body awareness. Relaxation is the single most beneficial thing you can learn to do for your health!

ANTIAGING TIP

Relaxation is a form of healing and rejuvenation. In this pose, we often struggle to relax, fighting tension in our bodies, fighting our impatience to get up, fighting our fast-moving thoughts. But with patience, determination, and concentration, you can teach yourself to enjoy the tranquility of Savasana and you will end each practice feeling fresh and revitalized.

Child's Pose

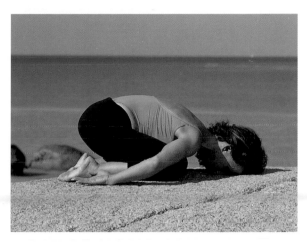

DIRECTIONS

| 1 | Kneel on the floor and bring your buttocks toward your heels. |

| 2 | Place your arms lengthwise, alongside your body. |

| 3 | Stretch your chin forward and gently lower your forehead to the floor, rounding your spine and shoulders. |

| 4 | Relax your neck muscles and relax into the pose. Hold the pose for 5 breaths. |

THE CLOCK IS STARTING TO REWIND

After the workout, ask yourself these questions:

- ○ Was it a good workout?

- ○ Do I feel toned and strong?

- ○ Do my thighs, legs, arms, and shoulders feel as if they were stretched?

- ○ Am I in sync and in balance?

- ○ Do I feel like I've just had a massage?

Give yourself time to enjoy every session. As you progress, you will grow from mimicking the illustrations and following the directions to gaining a deeper comprehension of the movements and postures. Your body will begin to set new stretching limits for itself. If you persevere, this workout will literally change your life and your physical and mental self-images. The benefits will resonate in every area of your life.

Practicing yoga is like breathing—it's never ending and constant. Stay true to yourself. You have the power!

ONE FINAL POSE

This pose is so beneficial and simple that you should incorporate it into your everyday life, rather than making it part of a routine you may do only a few days each week. I'm including it here so you can start benefiting from its antiaging properties right away.

Kegel Exercises

Kegel exercises work the perineal area and pelvic floor, increasing blood flow to the area. Practice them whenever possible, at any time of the day.

DIRECTIONS

1 Sit in a chair with your spine straight.

2 Contract the vaginal muscles as if you were holding back urination, and feel the pelvic floor being lifted up.

3 Hold the contraction for 5 breaths, and release. Repeat 5 to 10 times.

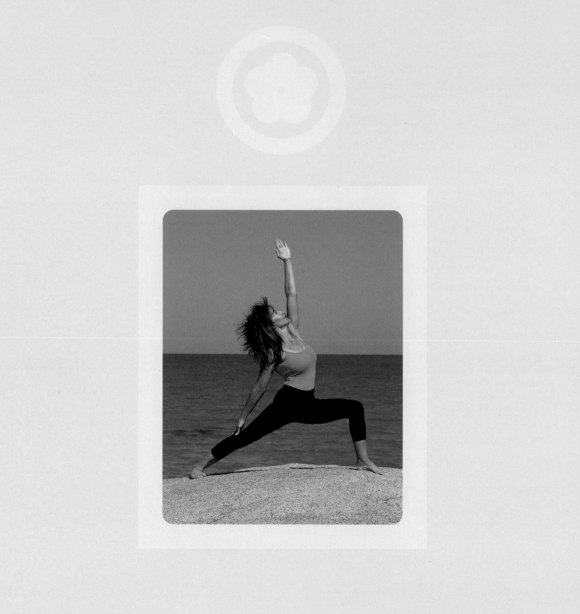

Chapter 4

Routine 2: Intermediate

Routine 2 is a little more challenging. It is a very effective strengthening, fat burning, and toning routine. In addition to these benefits, it also balances and nurtures your whole system, massaging and rejuvenating your internal organs. You'll see some poses you learned in Routine 1, such as Child's Pose, Cat's Pose, and Sun Salutation, before you're introduced to some new poses.

BALANCING POSES. Physically simple but mentally demanding, these improve your sense of balance and help develop concentration, patience, and determination. Physically, they firm your upper thighs; tighten your upper arms, hips, and buttocks; and improve the flexibility and strength of your lower spine and most of your body's muscles, giving you a youthful appearance.

EAGLE POSE. A balancing pose, as discussed above, but this one also improves the flexibility of your hips, knees, ankle joints, and shoulders.

KNEELING SIDE PLANK AND SIDE PLANK POSES. These poses build strength in your upper and lower body, giving you beautifully shaped arms and shoulders. They're great poses for building lean muscle.

LEG TONING POSES. These develop strong, lean, firm thighs, legs, and buttocks, and also lubricate your joints.

WARM DOWN STRETCHES. It is vitally important to stretch out and lengthen all the muscles you shorten and contract during the routine; flexibility is your reward for lengthening your shortened, contracted muscles. Standing Head to Knee Pose is used to immediately stretch and release your muscles after the Leg Toning Poses. The Butterfly and Open Angle Stretches lengthen the back side of the body, inner and outer thighs, and hamstrings. And the neck and shoulder stretches release those muscles that are so often neglected—and where stress so often manifests itself.

LYING DOWN SPINAL TWIST. This supported twist will unwind the stiffness of the spine and release tension buildup. It's a very soothing and calming pose.

ROUTINE 2

Child's Pose

Child's Pose is a resting pose. It is essential at the beginning, middle, and end of a practice session. When your muscles are contracted, lactic acid is produced as a result of a decrease in oxygen to your muscles. This causes fatigue. As your muscles relax, however, oxygen is immediately brought to them and lactic acid is reduced. Relaxing and resting even for a short time in the middle of any form of exercise will change your workout by making you more energized and by allowing your muscles time to recover.

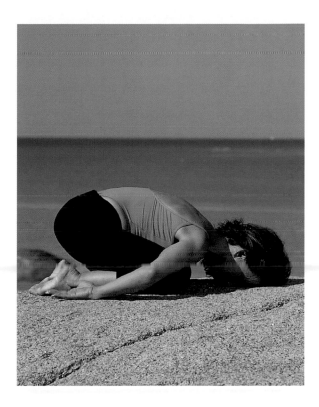

DIRECTIONS

1	Kneel on the floor and bring your buttocks toward your heels.
2	Place your arms lengthwise, alongside to your body.
3	Stretch your chin forward and gently lower your forehead to the floor, rounding your spine and shoulders.
4	Relax your neck muscles and relax into the pose. Hold the pose for 3 breaths.

✦ MODIFICATION

If your forehead does not touch the floor when your buttocks are close to your heels, open your knees slightly, allowing your forehead to touch the floor. Place a pillow under your head, if necessary, until you gain the necessary flexibility.

Cat's Pose

This pose warms up the spine and starts to create a little movement there.

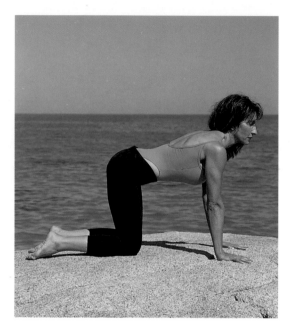 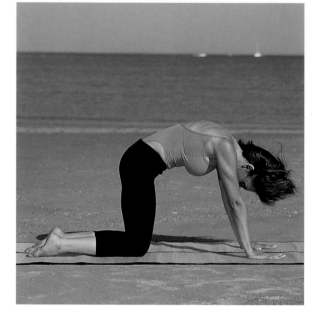

DIRECTIONS

1 Get on your hands and knees, with your palms under your shoulders and your knees under your hips.

2 Inhale, contract your abdominal muscles, and round your back, dropping your head toward the ground.

3 Exhale, release your abdominal muscles, arch your spine, and lift your head, sticking your buttocks out and up. All of the arching and rounding of your spine should initiate from your pelvis.

4 Repeat the pose 3 times.

From Cat's Pose, straighten your legs and raise your hips for the next pose, Downward Facing Dog.

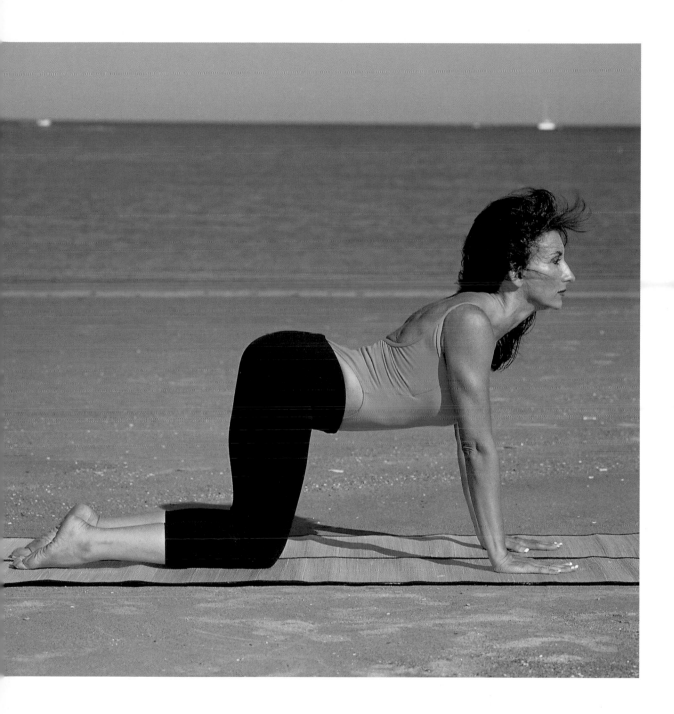

Downward Facing Dog

This pose will lengthen your spine as it stretches your entire back. Even though it's usually used as a resting pose, it is a powerful pose that is necessary to fully stretch out your back between the other poses. Think of a dog stretching when he wakes up from a nap, stretching his hips way up in the air as he lengthens his body. It looks good, and it feels great.

DIRECTIONS

1. From Cat's Pose, straighten your legs and shift your weight toward your heels and hips. Reach your arms as far forward as you can, and keep your hands and feet shoulder-width apart.

2. Spread your fingers open, and make sure the palms of your hands are pressing evenly onto the floor.

3. Lift your tailbone upwards, keeping your knees bent as necessary.

4. Shift your weight backwards toward your hips, and pull your shoulder blades back toward your waist. Your weight should be evenly distributed between your hands and your feet.

5. Drop your head toward the floor and consciously release your neck muscles. Hold the pose for 5 breaths.

CHALLENGE

As time progresses, try and straighten your legs and bring your heels toward the floor.

Stay in Downward Facing Dog until you begin the Forward Stretch.

DOWNWARD DOG POSE energizes and refreshes you in between postures. It strengthens the nerves and muscles in your upper body and legs, stretches the entire backside of your body, and increases blood supply to your head for clearer thinking.

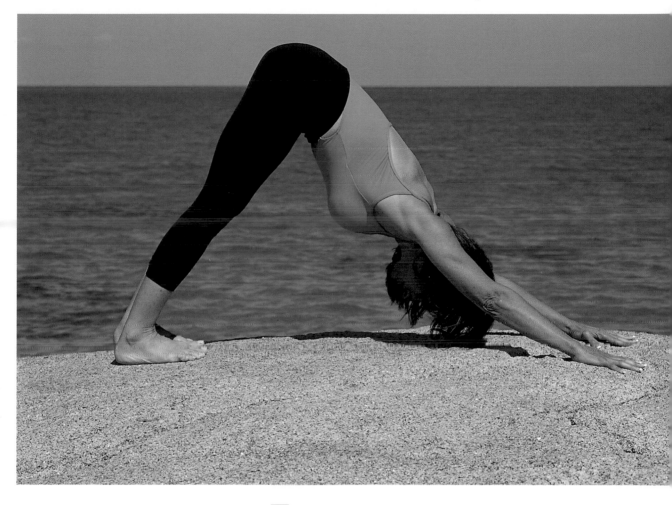

COMMON PROBLEMS

1. Not enough space between your hands and your legs.
2. Weight is not shifted backwards toward your hips and heels.
3. Hands aren't shoulder-width apart.
4. Feet aren't hip-width apart.

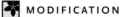 ### MODIFICATION

If you have wrist problems or carpal tunnel syndrome, buy a piece of spongy foam and cut a strip of it to the width of your yoga mat. Place this foam under the heels of your hands so that your wrists are slightly elevated. This will provide cushioning while shifting the weight away from your wrists and to the base of your palms. As you practice more, your wrists will get more flexible and the stiffness will ease, allowing you to stop using the foam support.

Three Warm-up Stretches:

Forward Stretch, Side Stretch, and Back Stretch

Always warm up with gentle stretching to prepare the body for more intense activity and reduce the risk of injury.

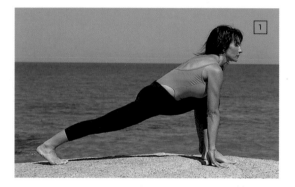

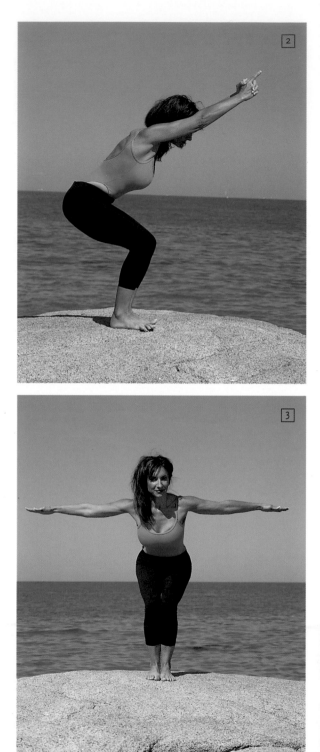

DIRECTIONS

1 Starting from Downward Facing Dog, raise your torso and bring your left foot in between your hands, then your right foot.

2 Keep your knees bent as you raise your torso and stretch your arms up and forward, for the Forward Stretch.

3   Holding your body in the same position, with knees still bent, stretch your arms all the way out to the side, for the Side Stretch.

4   Stretch your arms backwards toward your shoulders. Interlace your fingers and gently bend forward, straightening your legs as much as is comfortable, and releasing your head and neck muscles.

5   Stretch your arms a little higher away from your shoulders, for the Back Stretch. Hold for 3 breaths.

Slowly lift your torso to a standing position, still holding your hands and arms behind you, to prepare for the Lateral Side Stretch and Full Length Stretch.

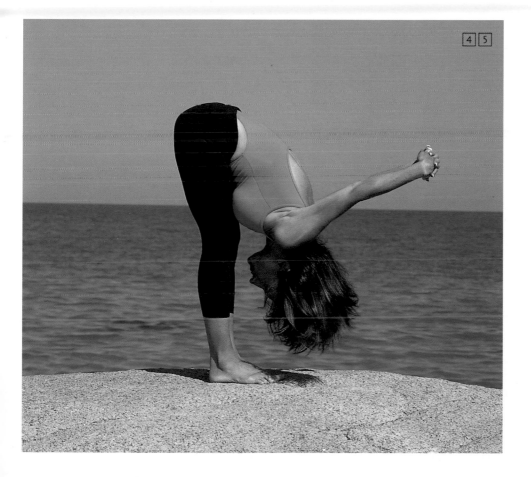

Lateral Side Stretch and Full Length Stretch

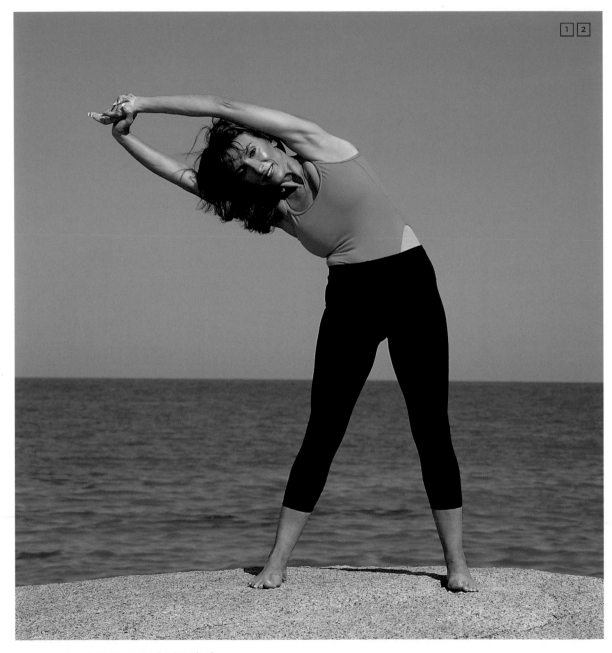

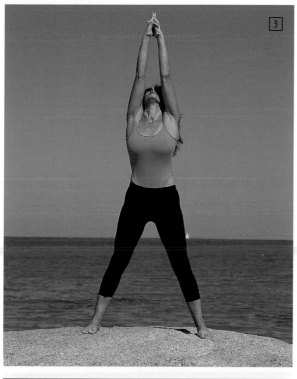

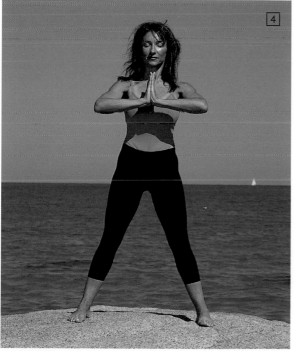

DIRECTIONS

1 Standing straight up, unclasp your hands and grab hold of your left wrist with your right hand. Stretch all the way over to the right.

2 Slowly return your body to standing straight, and switch hands, grabbing your right wrist with your left hand. Stretch all the way over to the left.

3 Slowly return your body to standing straight, release your hand, and interlace your fingers with your index fingers pointing upwards. Stretch your arms all the way over your head and gently release your head back. Feel the stretch from your waist all the way up to your pointed fingers.

4 Bring your hands to your heart center and close your eyes. Take 2 long, deep breaths, inhaling and exhaling completely, reaching down to the bottom part of your lungs.

Sun Salutation

Sun Salutations are made up of a series of poses, including standing poses, Plank, Chaturanga, Upward Facing Dog, and Downward Facing Dog. This series of poses awakens every inch of the body, imparting benefits to both the muscular and skeletal systems. Sun Salutations add suppleness to the spine, moving it in a backward and forward motion, and bring some flexibility to the shoulders, neck, arms, and hamstrings. They also jump-start the cardiovascular system through continuous movement of the body.

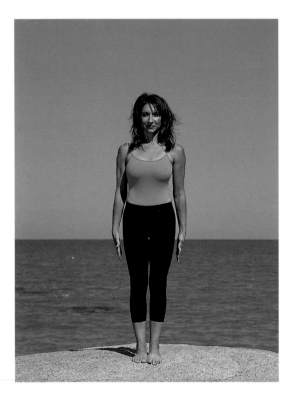
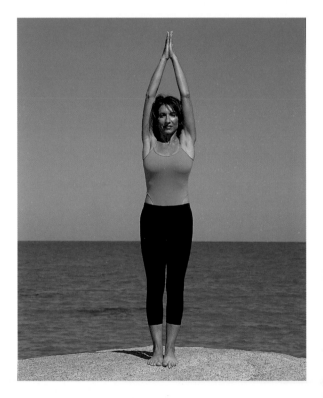

DIRECTIONS

1. Align your body, placing your feet together and your hands at your sides.

2. Inhale, roll your arms out with the palms facing out toward the ceiling, and bring your palms together overhead.

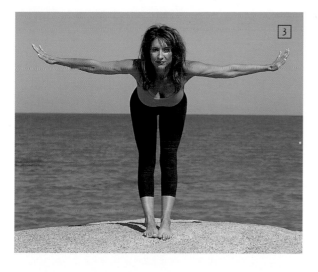

 3 Exhale, roll your arms out to the side and toward the floor, and gently release your head down toward the floor, lengthening your spine. Place your hands flat on the floor beside your feet.

4 Inhale and lift your head up.

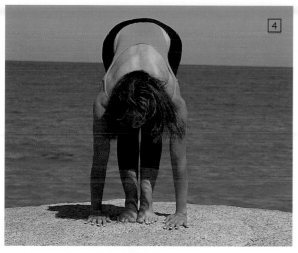

5 Exhale and release your head toward the floor.

Keep your hands on the floor and bring your right leg and then your left leg back, so your body is parallel to the floor and ready for Plank Pose.

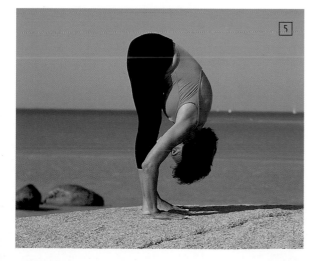

Plank Pose

(Sun Salutation, continued)

This is a weight-bearing pose. It will strengthen and prepare you for the other upper body poses that are more intense.

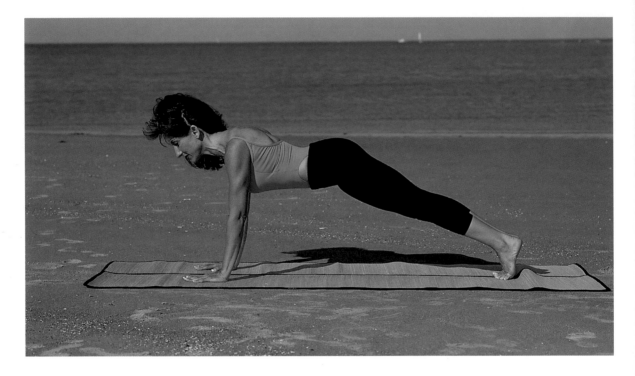

DIRECTIONS

1 Position your hands flat on the floor under your shoulders. Make sure they're pointing directly forward.

2 Tuck your toes under and come onto the balls of your feet, stretching through your heels.

3 Activate both thighs while keeping the back of your body really firm and flat.

4 Press firmly into your hands, and look toward the floor.

Continue directly into either the Modified Chaturanga or Challenge Chaturanga Pose.

Modified Chaturanga Pose

(Sun Salutation, continued)

Chaturanga is the Sanskrit term for a modified push-up. The pose will help you develop strength in your upper body and start to reshape your arms and shoulders.

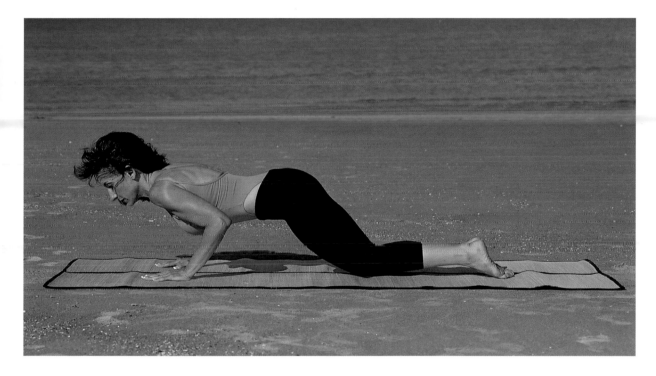

DIRECTIONS

1 Lower your knees to the floor, still keeping the muscles of your legs engaged.

2 Bend your elbows back, keeping them close to your body. Keep your shoulders square and gaze toward the floor.

3 Bend your elbows and bring your chest toward the floor, keeping your shoulders in line with your elbows, not lower, and keeping your body as straight a can be. Hold for 5 breaths.

Challenge Chaturanga Pose
(Sun Salutation, continued)

When you have sufficient strength, perform this pose in place of the Modified Chaturanga. This pose is used often, and needs special attention if you're going to master it.

DIRECTIONS

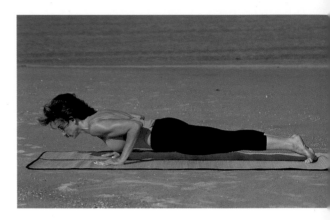

1 Remain in Plank Pose, with your knees off the floor.

2 Lower your upper body by bending your elbows, tucking them in, and hugging your ribcage. Continue to keep your body firm and supported; don't let it sag to the floor. If this happens, place your knees to the floor in Modified Chaturanga Pose.

3 Keep your elbows as close to your body as you can and your palms flat on the floor.

4 Lengthen your spine and keep your thighs active as you tighten your tummy muscles and gaze toward the floor. Hold the pose for 5 breaths.

COMMON PROBLEMS

1. Hands aren't directly under your shoulders.
2. Elbows aren't tucked in.
3. Not enough strength for Challenge Chaturanga.
4. Looking up, rather than gazing toward the floor.
5. Leading with your nose, rather than your chest, as you lower yourself toward the floor.
6. Allowing your shoulder blades to "cave in" toward each other.

From the Modified or Challenge Chaturanga, continue directly into Upward Facing Dog.

Upward Facing Dog
(Sun Salutation, continued)

This pose really starts to warm up the spine with a gentle backbend. It will also open your chest and strengthen your arms and shoulders.

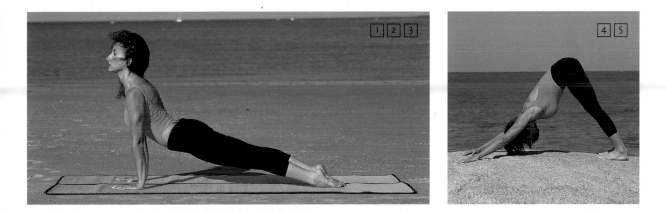

DIRECTIONS

1 From either Chaturanga Pose, scoop your chest and move your whole body forward and upward, rolling forward over the tops of your toes into Upward Facing Dog.

2 Open and lift your chest, straighten your arms, and lift your body so that only your hands and the tops of your feet support your body. Try and lift your thighs off the floor by tightening your thighs and buttocks.

3 Arch your spine and gaze directly in front of you, or gently drop your head back.

4 Curl your toes under, lift your hips, and stretch back into Downward Facing Dog.

5 Repeat the Sun Salutation series 2 or 3 times.

Standing Balancing and Toning Pose

DIRECTIONS

1. From a standing position, lift your arms out to your sides and bring your hands, palms together, to your heart center.

2. Find a focus point in front of you and keep your eyes on that one point.

3. Straighten your spine, and pull your abdominal muscles in.

4. Stretch your arms out to your sides at shoulder level and hold them there, using the muscles in your arms to point your fingers.

5. Lift your right knee in toward your chest, and flex your foot.

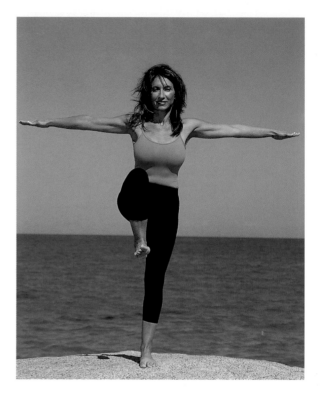

THE BALANCING POSTURE helps you develop concentration, and tones upper arms, upper thighs, and buttocks.

ANTIAGING TIP

This balancing posture increases circulation and strengthens the heart muscle, as well as improving mental, physical, and psychological powers.

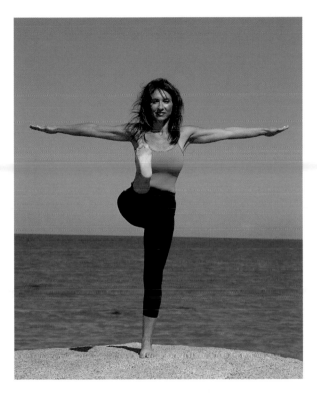

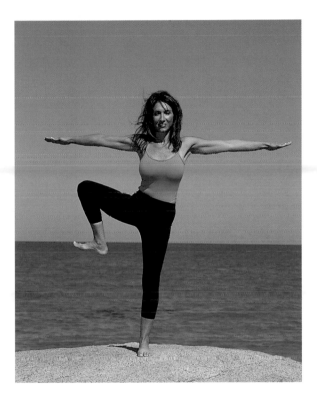

6 Straighten your leg forward, as straight as possible. Hold the pose for 5 breaths.

7 Bring your knee back in toward your chest, and smoothly open up your hip to the side. Keep your knee bent and your foot flexed.

Continued next page

Standing Balancing and Toning Pose (continued)

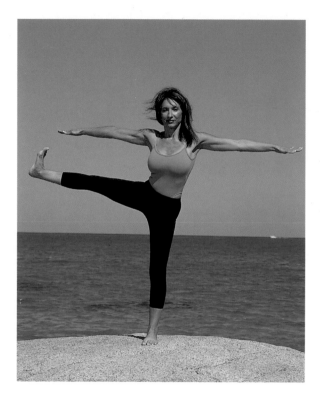

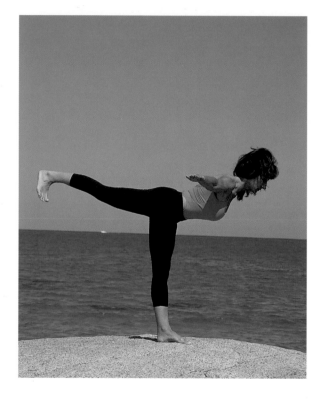

| 8 | Extend your leg out to the side. Hold for 5 breaths. |

| 9 | Bend your knee back in toward your chest. |

| 10 | Tip your body forward as you extend your leg out straight behind you. Extend through your heel, activating every muscle in your leg, and keep your hips squared. Your arms should still be stretched out, and your head, buttocks, and extended leg should be all in one straight line. |

| 11 | Gaze at one point on the floor. Hold the position for 5 to 10 breaths. |

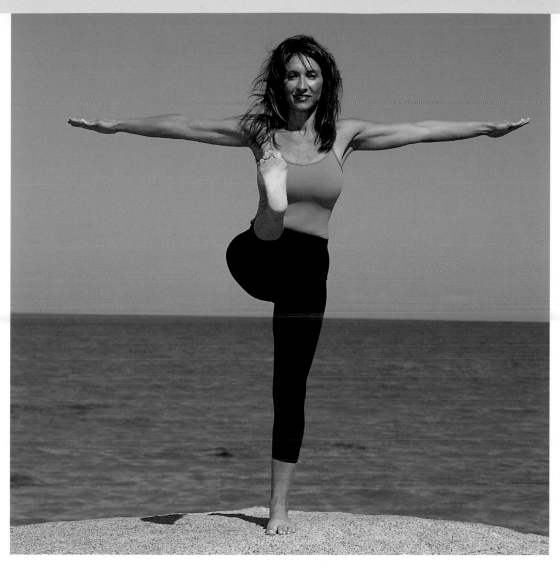

<table>
<tbody>
<tr><td>**12**</td><td>Slowly bring your torso up, still balancing on one leg.</td></tr>
</tbody>
</table>

12 Slowly bring your torso up, still balancing on one leg.

13 Bend your knee in and bring your leg forward as straight as you can, one more time. Hold for 5 breaths.

14 Repeat on the opposite leg.

CHALLENGE

Repeat the whole sequence twice on each leg.

COMMON PROBLEMS

1. Locking the knee when the leg is fully extended; always keep a soft knee to prevent injury.

2. Not tightening and fully engaging the muscles of your standing leg to steady and strengthen the ankle.

Eagle Pose

This is a great balancing pose. It requires concentration, stretching, and strengthening the shoulders and hips as you entwine your arms and your legs. It takes some time to develop enough flexibility to get deep into this posture, so you should modify the pose to suit your own strength and flexibility levels. You will gain benefits from this posture long before you can perform it perfectly.

DIRECTIONS

1 Stand tall, with your spine long and extended, your tummy tucked in, and your hips squared forward.

2 Inhale. Lift your left arm straight toward the ceiling. Wrap your right arm underneath your left arm and bend your elbows. Bring your hands together, holding your left thumb with your right hand, if possible.

3 Lift your elbows so they are in line with your shoulders.

4 Cross your right leg over your left, tucking your foot behind your calf muscle. If this is not possible, place your foot next to your calf muscle, or touch the toes of your foot to the floor.

5 Keep a straight spine as you exhale and slowly lower your body in a straight line, gazing at one point in front of you. Hold the pose for 10 breaths. Make sure you breathe evenly, allowing your shoulders and hips to expand.

6 Repeat the pose, balancing on the opposite leg.

CHALLENGE
Repeat Eagle Pose twice.

COMMON PROBLEMS
1. Leaning forward instead of holding your head and spine in a straight line.
2. Twisting to the side, instead of keeping your elbows and knees in a straight line.
3. Allowing the standing knee to twist so it is not facing forward.

Eagle Pose supplies fresh blood to the kidneys

and sexual organs for increased sexuality.

THE EAGLE POSE, a balancing pose, helps you to develop physical and mental equilibrium, releases tension in your upper back and hips, and increases flexibility in your ankles and knees.

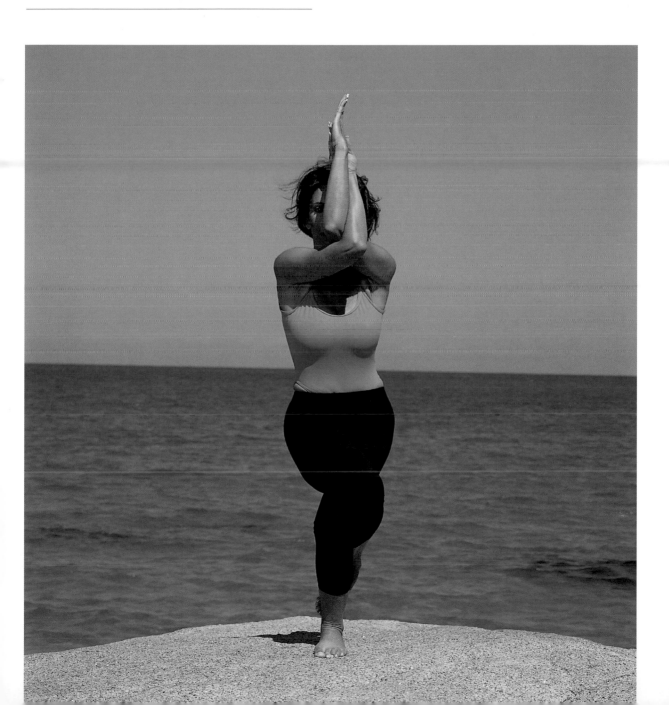

Sun Salutation

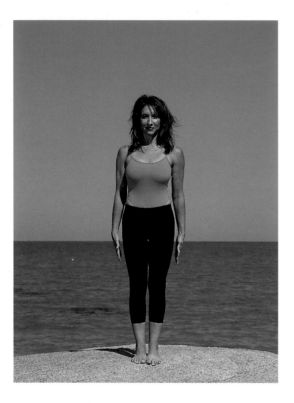 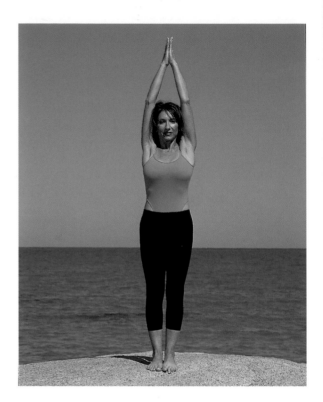

DIRECTIONS

1 Align your body, placing your feet together and your hands at your sides.

2 Inhale, roll your arms out with the palms facing out toward the ceiling, and bring your palms together overhead.

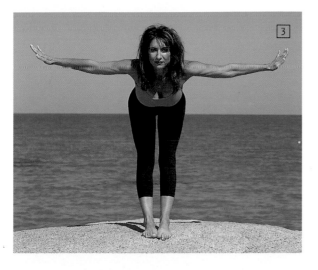

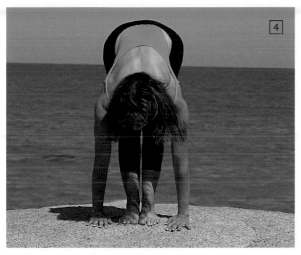

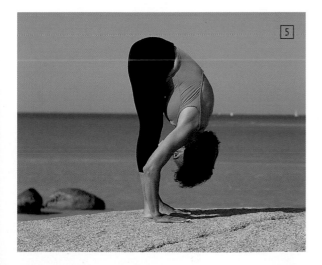

3 Exhale, roll your arms out to the side and toward the floor, and gently release your head down toward the floor, lengthening your spine. Place your hands flat on the floor beside your feet.

4 Inhale and lift your head up.

5 Exhale and release your head toward the floor.

Keep your hands on the floor and bring your right leg and then your left leg back, so your body is parallel to the floor and ready for Plank Pose.

Plank Pose
(Sun Salutation, continued)

This is a weight-bearing pose. It will strengthen and prepare you for the other upper body poses that are more intense.

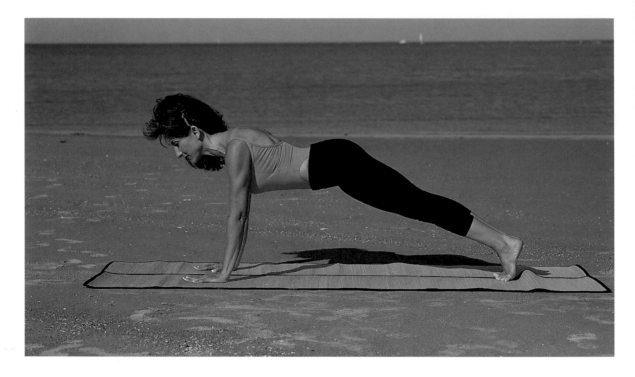

DIRECTIONS

1 Position your hands flat on the floor under your shoulders. Make sure they're pointing directly forward.

2 Tuck your toes under and come onto the balls of your feet, stretching through your heels.

3 Activate both thighs while keeping the back of your body really firm and flat.

4 Press firmly into your hands, and look toward the floor.

Continue directly into either the Modified Chaturanga or Challenge Chaturanga Pose.

Modified Chaturanga Pose

(Sun Salutation, continued)

Chaturanga is the Sanskrit term for a modified push-up. The pose will help you develop strength in your upper body and start to reshape your arms and shoulders.

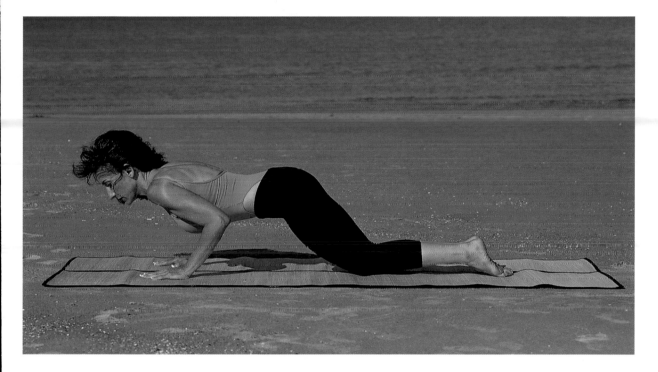

DIRECTIONS

1 Lower your knees to the floor, still keeping the muscles of your legs engaged.

2 Bend your elbows back, keeping them close to your body. Keep your shoulders square and gaze toward the floor.

3 Bend your elbows and bring your chest toward the floor, keeping your shoulders in line with your elbows, not lower, and keeping your body as straight a can be. Hold for 5 breaths.

Challenge Chaturanga Pose

(Sun Salutation, continued)

When you have sufficient strength, perform this pose in place of the Modified Chaturanga. This pose is used often, and needs special attention if you're going to master it.

DIRECTIONS

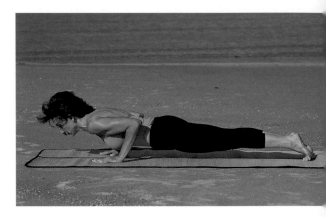

1	Remain in Plank Pose, with your knees off the floor.

2	Lower your upper body by bending your elbows, tucking them in, and hugging your ribcage. Continue to keep your body firm and supported; don't let it sag to the floor. If this happens, place your knees to the floor in Modified Chaturanga Pose.

3	Keep your elbows as close to your body as you can and your palms flat on the floor.

4	Lengthen your spine and keep your thighs active as you tighten your tummy muscles and gaze toward the floor. Hold the pose for 5 breaths.

COMMON PROBLEMS

1. Hands aren't directly under your shoulders.
2. Elbows aren't tucked in.
3. Not enough strength for Challenge Chaturanga.
4. Looking up, rather than gazing toward the floor.
5. Leading with your nose, rather than your chest, as you lower yourself toward the floor.
6. Allowing your shoulder blades to "cave in" toward each other.

From the Modified or Challenge Chaturanga, continue directly into Upward Facing Dog.

Upward Facing Dog

Sun Salutation, continued

This pose really starts to warm up the spine with a gentle backbend. It will also open your chest and strengthen your arms and shoulders.

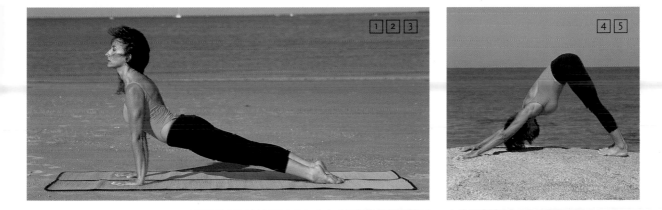

DIRECTIONS

1 From either Chaturanga Pose, scoop your chest and move your whole body forward and upward, rolling forward over the tops of your toes into Upward Facing Dog.

2 Open and lift your chest, straighten your arms, and lift your body so that only your hands and the tops of your feet support your body. Try and lift your thighs off the floor by tightening your thighs and buttocks.

3 Arch your spine and gaze directly in front of you, or gently drop your head back.

4 Curl your toes under, lift your hips, and stretch back into Downward Facing Dog, transferring your weight back towards your heels.

5 Repeat the Sun Salutation series 2 or 3 times.

Stay in Downward Facing Dog until you begin the Kneeling Side Plank or Side Plank Pose.

Kneeling Side Plank Pose

This is a very powerful strengthening and toning arm and shoulder pose. It will help you develop tremendous strength in your upper body.

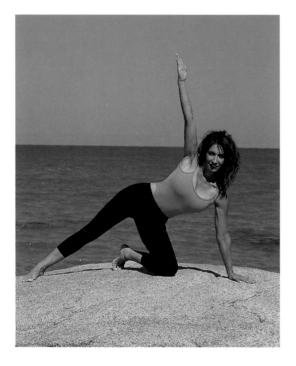

THE KNEELING SIDE PLANK POSE reshapes your three major arm and shoulder muscles, tones your legs, and helps you develop coordination.

DIRECTIONS

1 From Downward Facing Dog, bring your left knee to the ground and balance on your left hand and left knee, turning the body to face sideways.

2 Inhale and raise your right arm, stretched to the ceiling, opening your shoulder and your chest.

3 Move your shoulders away from your ears, lengthening your spine and creating space. Look toward your upper hand or, if you have neck problems, in front of you or to the floor.

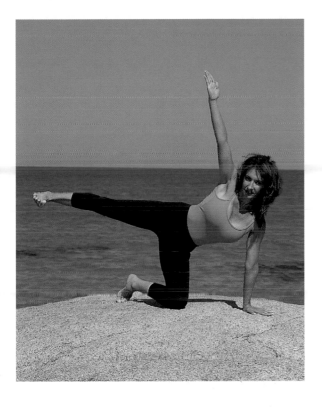

4 Exhale, and lift your right foot off the floor until it is in line with your hip. Flex your foot, extend through your heel, and work every muscle in your leg as you continue to lengthen your leg away from your hip. Hold the pose for 5 breaths.

5 Repeat the pose with the opposite leg.

COMMON PROBLEMS

1. Allowing your wrist to support your weight. Activate all the muscles in the body to prevent this.
2. Letting the body sink into the shoulder and neck. Always lengthen and extend outwards while in this pose.
3. Problem knees—if you have them, place some kind of cushioning under your knees before you begin the pose.

ANTIAGING TIP

Arms and shoulders are extensively exercised in this pose, firming sagging, loose arm skin and giving you a more youthful appearance.

Side Plank Pose

In this pose, both your knees are off the floor for more intense strengthening and toning.

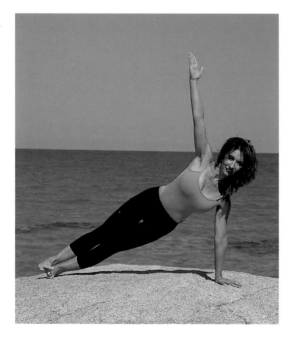

THE SIDE PLANK POSE is a more intense version of the kneeling side plank pose, providing very visible results.

DIRECTIONS

 1 From Downward Facing Dog, transition into Plank Pose.

2 Roll to your left side, balancing on your feet, so your inner thighs are touching.

3 Bring your right hand up, pointing toward the ceiling. Your lower hand should be directly under your shoulder. Look to the ceiling or in front of you.

ANTIAGING TIP

This pose will super-strengthen the entire body, for increased power and stamina.

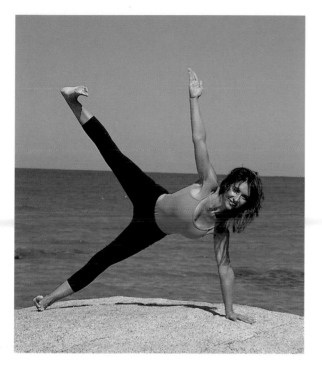

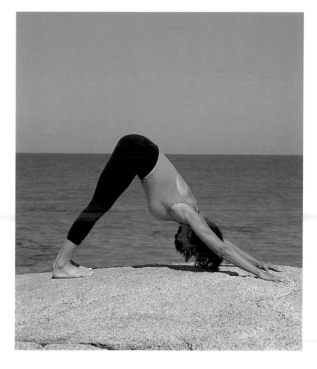

4 Your upper hip should be directly in line with your lower hip, and your heels, hips, and shoulders should be in one line.

5 Lift your right foot off the floor, keeping your foot flexed. Extend through the heel, and lengthen your leg away from your hip.

6 You can gaze up, in front of you, or toward the ground. Hold the pose for 5 breaths.

7 Repeat the pose on the opposite side.

Release your knee or knees back to the floor and get onto all fours. Stretch back into Downward Facing Dog for 3 breaths to prepare for the Leg Toning Poses.

MODIFICATION

If your arm starts to wobble, lower your knee to the floor. Keep working the Kneeling Side Plank Pose to gain strength.

Leg Toning Poses

These toning exercises for the legs and buttocks are simple yet powerful. To get the full benefit of these poses, keep the muscles of your thighs and buttocks tightly squeezed throughout.

DIRECTIONS

1 From Downward Facing Dog, bring your left foot between your hands and spread your legs about 3 feet apart.

2 Turn your right foot out at a 45-degree angle.

3 Bend your front knee at a 90-degree angle.

4 Extend your torso forward, keeping your chest just off your thigh, and reach forward with your arms. Interlace your fingers and place your head between your arms. Hold the pose for 5 breaths.

5 Keeping your legs and torso in the same position, bring your arms back behind you, like wings. Hold the pose for 5 breaths.

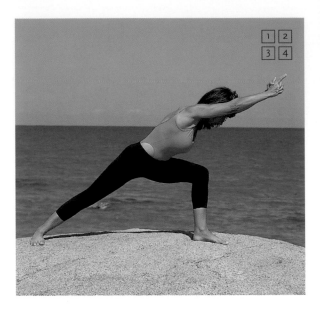

THE LEG TONING POSES reshape your legs, are great for balance, and add a cardiovascular element to your workout.

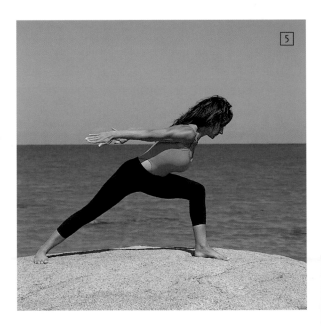

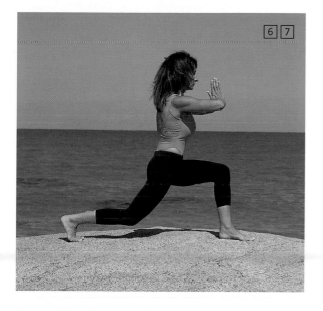

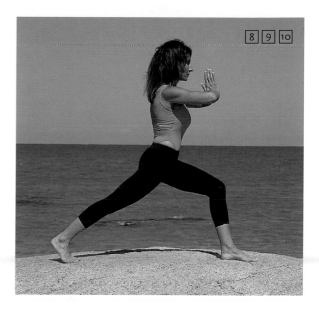

6. Keeping your legs and torso in the same position, bring your arms back in front of you, as in Step 4. Hold the pose for 5 breaths.

7. Bring your hands to your heart center. Keeping your spine straight, lift your right heel off the floor and extend your right leg as straight as can be.

8. Bend your left knee and slowly lower yourself toward the floor. Hold the pose for 5 breaths.

9. Slowly raise your body back up until your back leg is straight. Hold the pose for 5 breaths. Repeat two or more times.

10. Repeat the whole sequence on the opposite leg.

ANTIAGING TIP

This pose will strengthen and tone the rectus femoris and abductor muscles of the thigh, as well as the gluteus maximus of the buttocks. The expression "Use it or lose it" rings true here—these muscles can get toned and reshaped at any age.

Standing Head to Knee Pose

This pose is actually a forward bend. It seriously stretches out the hamstrings and contracted leg and thigh muscles, one leg at a time.

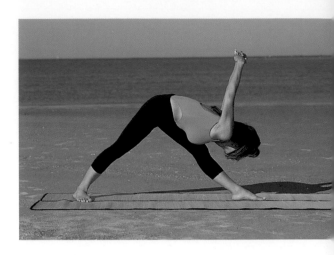

THE STANDING HEAD-TO-KNEE POSE is an excellent all-over body stretch that lengthens your legs, hips, and entire backside.

DIRECTIONS

1 From the Leg Toning Pose, lower your back heel so your foot is flat on the floor and turned out at a 45-degree angle. Your front toe should be facing forward, and both your legs should be straight, thighs active.

2 Square your hips and shoulders forward, interlace your hands behind your back, and draw your arms over your head, as high as possible.

3 Inhale, and lengthen through your entire spine, from your tailbone to your head.

4 Exhale, and bend your body forward from your hips. Lift your tailbone up toward the ceiling, leading with your chest toward your leg, and surrender your head toward the floor. Release your neck muscles, keeping them soft. Keep your elbows straight as your arms are lifted, and keep your head and spine in a straight line. Hold the pose for 5 breaths.

5 Repeat the pose on the opposite leg.

MODIFICATION

If interlacing your hands behind your back is too much of a challenge at first, begin performing this pose with your hands on your waist, instead.

COMMON PROBLEMS

1. Leading with the head and not your chest.
2. Not lengthening your spine as you fold forward.

Butterfly Stretch

This is an incredible hip opener. It also opens and stretches the groin area.

DIRECTIONS

1 Sit with your knees bent and the soles of your feet together. Lift your chest upward.

2 Grasp your feet with both hands and bring them in as close to your body as you can.

3 Keeping your back straight, slowly lower your chest toward the floor. Keep your chin forward and your knees as close to the floor as possible. Hold the pose for 5 breaths.

CHALLENGE

Hold the butterfly stretch for 10 breaths

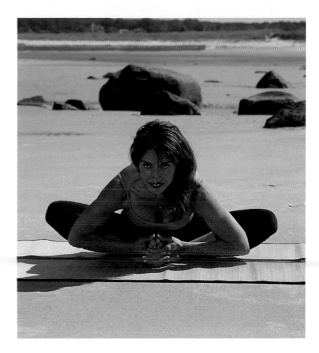

THE BUTTERFLY STRETCH increases mobility of your hips, lower back and groin, and improves the health of your pelvic region.

ANTIAGING TIP

This pose is excellent for the health of the pelvic region, increasing the blood supply to that area.

Open Angle Stretch

You'll reap tremendous benefits from the intense hamstring stretch this pose provides. You'll also stretch your inner legs and open your hips and groin. And as you stretch forward and then to the sides, you'll gain flexibility in your spine.

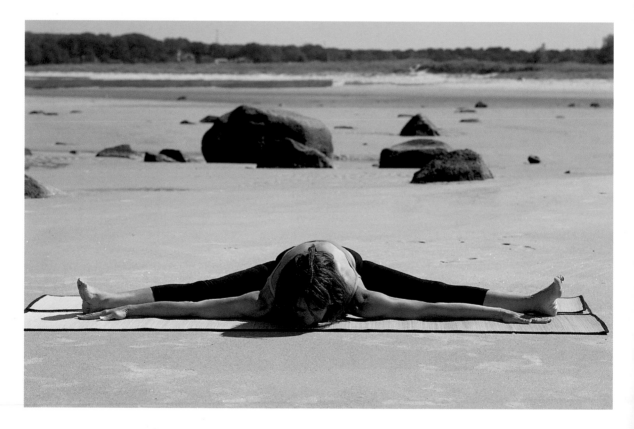

THE OPEN ANGLE POSE stretches your inner thighs and groin, which is excellent for female reproductive organs.

DIRECTIONS

1 Spread your legs wide apart and press your hamstrings and calf muscles to the floor. Flex your feet and sit tall.

2 Stretch your arms over your head, lengthening your spine, and bend from the waist. When your hands touch the ground, gently walk them forward until you feel a good stretch. Ultimately you want to reach final position, where your chest and chin rest on the floor and your arms are extended all the way to each side.

3 Make sure your spine stays long and extended, and be conscious of releasing your neck muscles. Hold the pose for 5 breaths.

4 For an extra stretch, crawl your torso toward your right leg and walk your hands as far forward as you can, reaching for your right foot. Hold the pose for 5 breaths, then repeat with your left leg.

Return to the pose's starting position and prepare for the Lateral Torso Stretch.

CHALLENGE
Hold the pose for 10 breaths.

MODIFICATION
Sit on the edge of a folded blanket and wrap a towel or strap around each leg. Hold them there with your arms extended, and tilt your pelvis forward, being careful not to round your back.

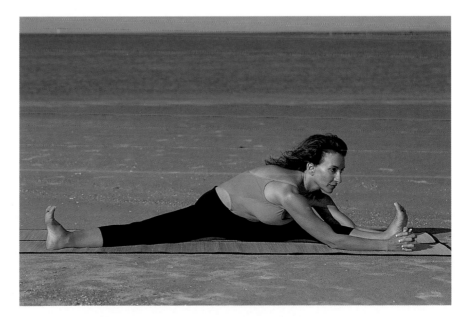

Lateral Torso Stretch

This pose starts in the same position as Open Angle Pose, but extends your body all the way to each side, giving your waist and spine a good, strong stretch.

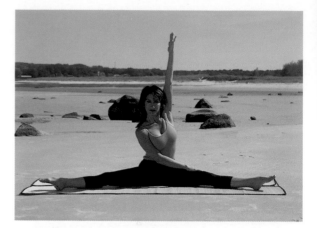

DIRECTIONS

| 1 | With your legs spread wide and your hamstring and calf muscles pressed to the floor, grab your left thigh with your right hand and extend your left arm toward the ceiling. |

| 2 | Bring your right shoulder toward your right thigh, leaning over to get a wonderful stretch to the side of the waist. Hold for 5 breaths. |

| 3 | Repeat the pose to the other side. |

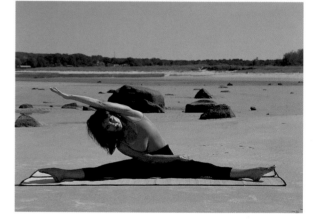

THE LATERAL TORSO STRETCH works your inner thighs, torso, hips, and pelvic muscles.

ANTIAGING TIP

This pose is excellent for the health of the pelvic region; it will give you a healthy prostate and reproductive organs at any age.

Arm and Shoulder Stretch

(Stretch I)

This exercise and the Neck and Shoulder Stretch take the tension out of tight neck and shoulder muscles.

DIRECTIONS

1 Sit on your knees, buttocks to heels. (If this is hard on your knees, use padding or a towel, or fold over your mat; if this is still uncomfortable, perform the pose from a standing position.)

2 With your spine erect, raise your left arm over your head and bend your right arm behind your back, and clasp your hands. (If your hands do not meet behind your back, use a small towel to bridge the gap, and walk your hands toward each other.)

3 Make sure your shoulders are level and your collarbones are broad. Hold the pose for 10 breaths.

4 Switch arms and repeat the pose.

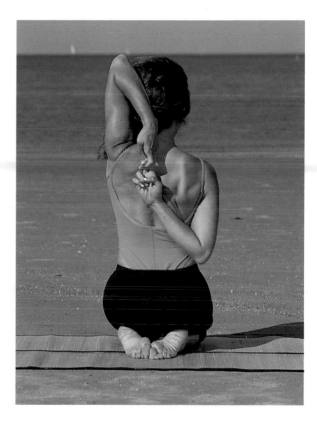

THE ARM AND SHOULDER STRETCH POSE I releases upper shoulder and back tension, increases flexibility, and improves posture by opening your chest.

ANTIAGING TIP

This pose and the one that follows loosen tight shoulder joints, improving posture and straightening rounded shoulders, for a more youthful appearance.

Neck and Shoulder Stretch
(Stretch II)

THE NECK AND SHOULDER POSE II releases tension from your shoulders, upper back, and rotator cuff, as well as strengthens your neck and shoulders.

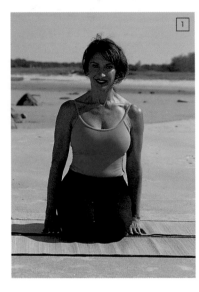 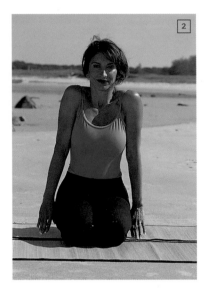 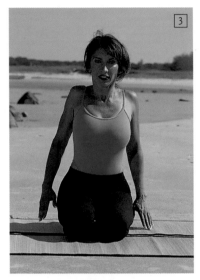

DIRECTIONS

1 Sit on your knees, buttocks to heels. Pull your shoulders back and down, and rest your arms next to your body.

2 Lift your shoulders toward your ears.

3 Rotate your shoulders backwards in a little circle, bringing them back to their original position. Repeat this shoulder roll 5 times.

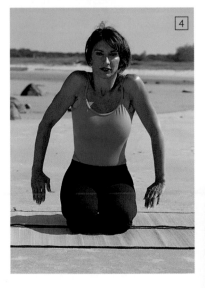

4 Rotate your shoulders forward in little circles, bringing them back to their original position. Repeat this shoulder roll 5 times.

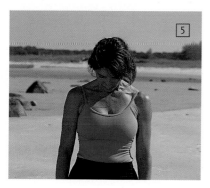

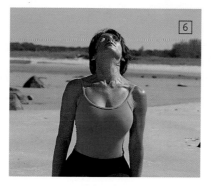

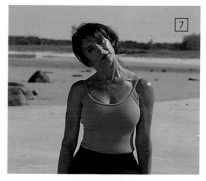

5 Gently lower your chin toward your chest, stretching the back of your neck.

6 Gently lower your head as far back as you can without pain, stretching the front side of your neck. Bring your head back up to starting position.

7 Gently lower your head to the right, holding your shoulders away from your ears. Repeat to the other side.

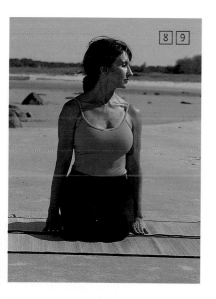

8 Return your head to the center. Turn your head to the right, keeping your head level, and look over your right shoulder as far as you can comfortably. Turn your head back to the center, and repeat on the other side.

9 Close your eyes and sit for a few breaths before moving to the next pose.

ANTIAGING TIP

Twisting to look behind you gets harder as you get older, so massaged, released shoulder and neck muscles make a difference in everything we do. More than just contributing to a youthful appearance, they're essential for safe driving, when you need to be able to look behind you.

Lying Down Spinal Twist

This twist is relaxing and easy to practice. It's simple and gentle, yet entirely stretches the muscles in your back and hips. This posture is wonderful to use near the end of the routine to release the muscles in your lower back.

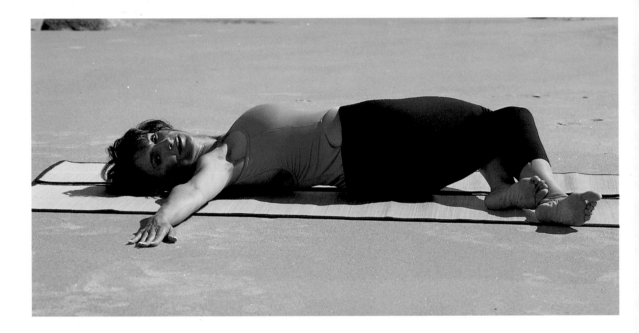

DIRECTIONS

1 Lie flat on the floor, arms stretched out to the side and palms pressing into the floor.

2 Inhale, bend your left leg and wrap your right thigh over your left thigh, entwining your legs and keeping your back on the floor.

3 Exhale and bring your legs over to the left, twisting your spine to the right as you turn your head to the right.

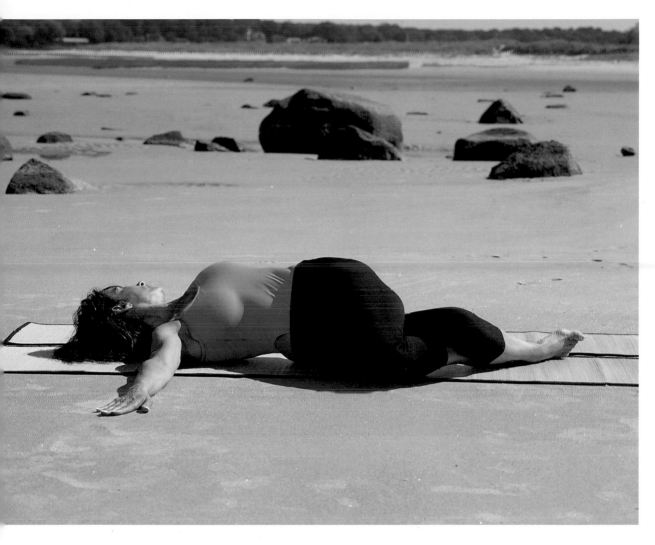

4 Slowly bring your legs back to the center, uncross and recross your legs the opposite way, and repeat the pose to the opposite side.

THE LYING DOWN SPINAL TWIST tones your abs and relieves lower back pain caused by muscular tension.

ANTIAGING TIP

Whether you are very active or more sedentary, everyday life causes a lot of abuse to the spine. This gentle twist helps your spine recuperate.

Savasana, or Corpse Pose

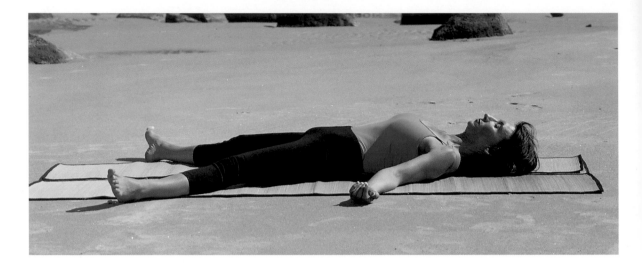

DIRECTIONS

1 Lie flat on your back with your feet apart and your toes relaxed and facing out.

2 Place your arms slightly out from your sides, with your palms up.

3 Close your eyes and consciously release and relax each and every muscle, transferring all the weight of your body to the floor.

4 Slowly bring your focus to your breath, and feel the rhythmic movement of your body as you breathe in and out. Really get in touch with your body and your breath, holding the pose for 5 to 10 minutes.

5 Wrap your arms around your knees, drawing them into your chest, and roll to your right side into a fetal position.

From this position, roll onto your knees to prepare for Child's Pose.

 MODIFICATION

If your lower back feels uncomfortable lying in Savasana, bend your knees instead of straightening your legs.

Child's Pose

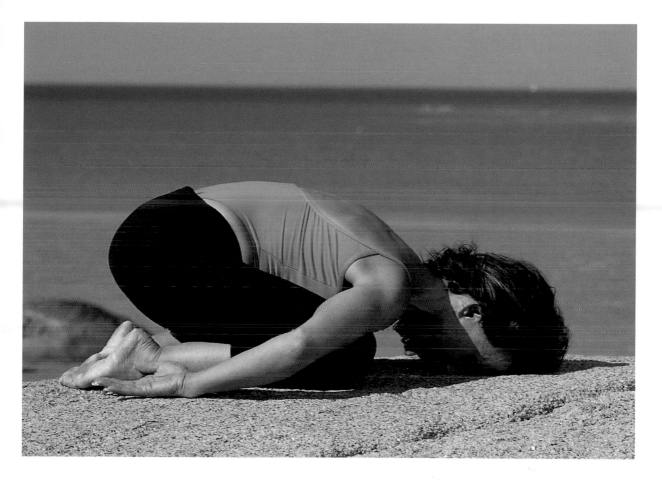

DIRECTIONS

1 Kneel on the floor and bring your buttocks toward your heels.

2 Place your arms lengthwise, alongside to your body.

3 Stretch your chin forward and gently lower your forehead to the floor, rounding your spine and shoulders.

4 Relax your neck muscles and relax into the pose. Hold the pose for 5 breaths.

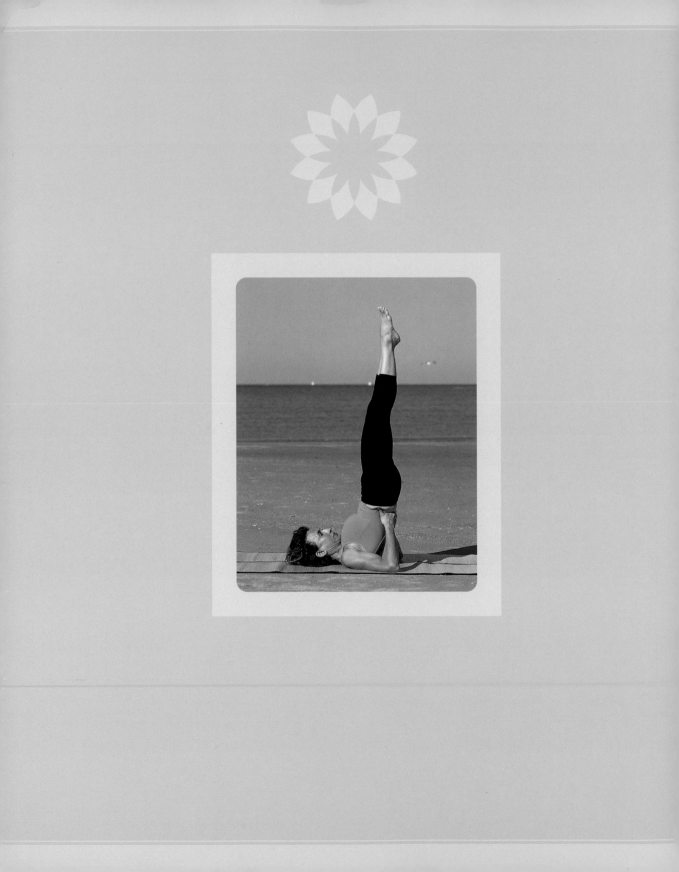

Chapter 5

Routine 3: Advanced

All three routines follow the same format, so you'll get used to performing the poses with variations. Eventually you'll be able to flow beautifully from one pose to another, as we do in class, just by seeing the names of the poses. It is then that you'll reap all the benefits that yoga has to offer.

In Routine 3, we concentrate on backbends, forward bends, and abdominal strengthening. As before, we begin with the warm-up poses, but in this routine we take the backbends a step further, incorporating them into the Sun Salutation. The intention here is to feel like your body is completely liquid, agile, and youthful. We all want to experience that full range of movement, especially as we get older.

To prevent injury, the body really needs to be warmed up before you practice any backbend. Never force a backbend if you are stiff; always ease into the pose gently and have patience. The amount you can stretch will grow in increments, and every extra inch of movement is an improvement. Forward bends flex the spine and backbends extend it, stimulating and strengthening circulation and respiration, both of which are fundamental to good health.

SEATED FORWARD BEND. This pose is absolutely necessary to counterbalance the backbends. This simple but powerful pose folds the body almost in half, giving a comprehensive stretch to the entire back of the body.

INCLINED PLANE. This complements the Seated Forward Bend, strengthens shoulders, arms, and hips, and increases their flexibility and muscle coordination.

ABDOMINALS. The routine in this book, although relatively simple, is dynamic and works wonders for strengthening abdominal muscles. Really follow the directions, and build up to more repetitions as you build strength. Strong abs are powerfully youthful, and in balance with a strong back, they will help you feel more powerful in your everyday life.

SPINAL BALANCING AND HIP ROTATION, AND DOLPHIN WITH LEG AND BUTTOCKS TONING POSE. These postures have strong antiaging effects because they build strength, increase the range of motion in your hips, and firm your thighs, buttocks, and upper body.

OPEN ANGLE POSE AND LATERAL TORSO STRETCH. This stretch is wonderful for tight hamstrings resulting from too much or too little activity. Work with the modifications suggested, and over time and with practice the hamstrings will release. Improving circulation to the reproductive organs and stimulating the ovaries and prostate gland, this pose increases blood to these organs for a healthier and more active sex life.

SHOULDER STAND. It's called the "Queen of poses," simply because the whole body benefits from it. Because it is an inverted pose, your heart and brain receive a healthy rush of oxygenated blood. It boosts the circulatory system and as a result has fatigue-relieving properties. When you are standing, your body has to work against gravity to pump blood from the lower extremities back to your heart; the Shoulder Stand is invaluable because it reverses gravity.

ROUTINE 3

Child's Pose

Child's Pose is a resting pose. It is essential at the beginning, middle, and end of a practice session. When your muscles are contracted, lactic acid is produced as a result of a decrease in oxygen to your muscles. This causes fatigue. As your muscles relax, however, oxygen is immediately brought to them and lactic acid is reduced. Relaxing and resting even for a short time in the middle of any form of exercise will change your workout by making you more energized and by allowing your muscles time to recover.

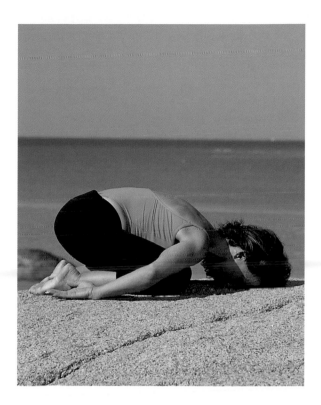

DIRECTIONS

1	Kneel on the floor and bring your buttocks toward your heels.
2	Place your arms lengthwise, alongside to your body.
3	Stretch your chin forward and gently lower your forehead to the floor, rounding your spine and shoulders.
4	Relax your neck muscles and relax into the pose. Hold the pose for 3 breaths.

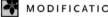 MODIFICATION

If your forehead does not touch the floor when your buttocks are close to your heels, open your knees slightly, allowing your forehead to touch the floor. Place a pillow under your head, if necessary, until you gain the necessary flexibility.

Cat's Pose

This pose warms up the spine and starts to create a little movement there.

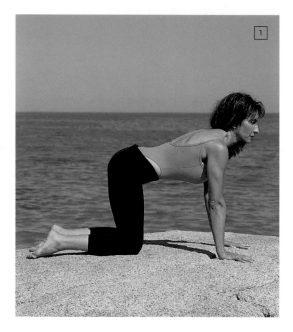 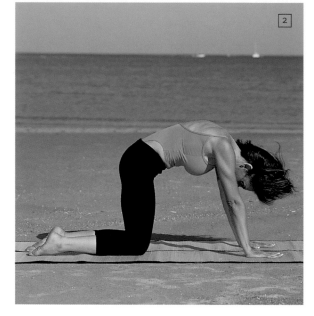

DIRECTIONS

1 Get on your hands and knees, with your palms under your shoulders and your knees under your hips.

2 Inhale, contract your abdominal muscles, and round your back, dropping your head toward the ground.

3 Exhale, release your abdominal muscles, arch your spine, and lift your head, sticking your buttocks out and up. All of the arching and rounding of your spine should initiate from your pelvis.

4 Repeat the pose 3 times.

From Cat's Pose, straighten your legs and raise your hips for the next pose, Downward Facing Dog.

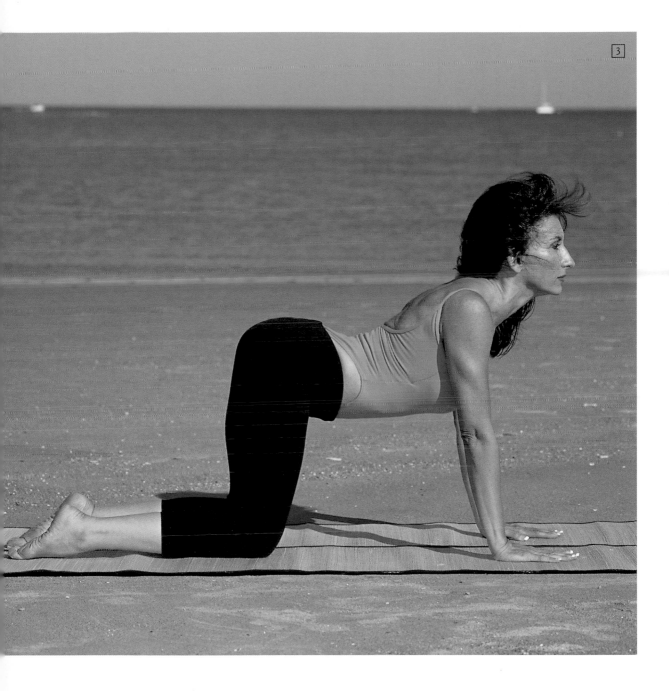

Downward Facing Dog

This pose will lengthen your spine as it stretches your entire back. Even though it's usually used as a resting pose, it is a powerful pose that is necessary to fully stretch out your back between the other poses. Think of a dog stretching when he wakes up from a nap, stretching his hips way up in the air as he lengthens his body. It looks good, and it feels great.

DIRECTIONS

1 From Cat's Pose, straighten your legs and shift your weight toward your heels and hips. Reach your arms as far forward as you can, and keep your hands and feet shoulder-width apart.

2 Spread your fingers open, and make sure the palms of your hands are pressing evenly onto the floor.

3 Lift your tailbone upwards, keeping your knees bent as necessary.

4 Shift your weight backwards toward your hips, and pull your shoulder blades back toward your waist. Your weight should be evenly distributed between your hands and your feet.

5 Drop your head toward the floor and consciously release your neck muscles. Hold the pose for 5 breaths.

CHALLENGE

As time progresses, try and straighten your legs and bring your heels toward the floor.

Stay in Downward Facing Dog until you begin the Forward Stretch.

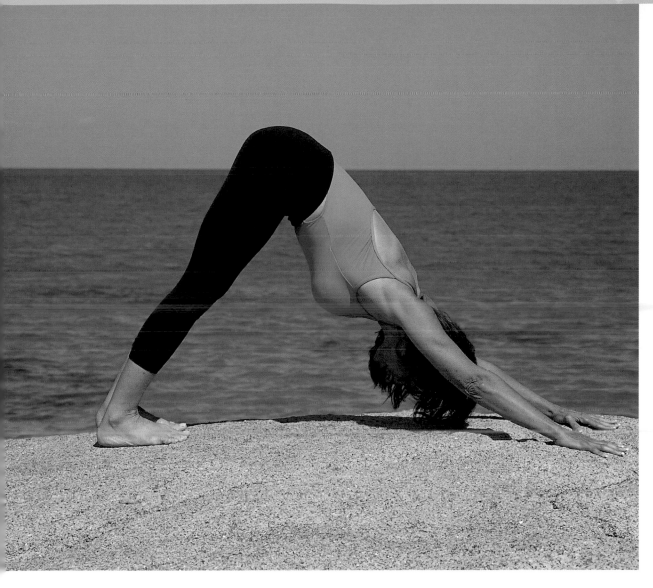

COMMON PROBLEMS

1. Not enough space between your hands and your legs.
2. Weight is not shifted backwards toward your hips and heels.
3. Hands aren't shoulder-width apart.
4. Feet aren't hip-width apart.

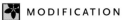 **MODIFICATION**

If you have wrist problems or carpal tunnel syndrome, buy a piece of spongy foam and cut a strip of it to the width of your yoga mat. Place this foam under the heels of your hands so that your wrists are slightly elevated. This will provide cushioning while shifting the weight away from your wrists and to the base of your palms. As you practice more, your wrists will get more flexible and the stiffness will ease, allowing you to stop using the foam support.

Three Warm-up Stretches:

Forward Stretch,
Side Stretch, and Back Stretch

Always warm up with gentle stretching to prepare the body for more intense activity and reduce the risk of injury.

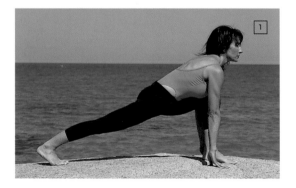

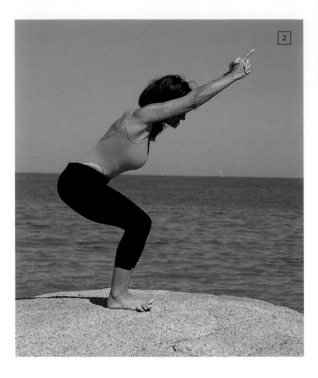

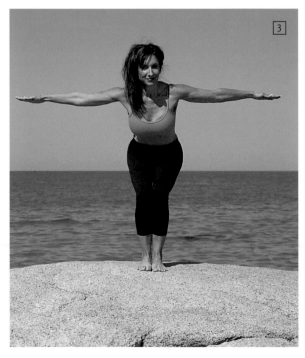

DIRECTIONS

1 Starting from Downward Facing Dog, raise your torso and bring your left foot in between your hands, then your right foot.

2 Keep your knees bent as you raise your torso and stretch your arms up and forward, for the Forward Stretch.

3 Holding your body in the same position, with knees still bent, stretch your arms all the way out to the side, for the Side Stretch.

4 Stretch your arms backwards toward your shoulders. Interlace your fingers and gently bend forward, straightening your legs as much as is comfortable, and releasing your head and neck muscles.

5 Stretch your arms a little higher away from your shoulders, for the Back Stretch. Hold for 3 breaths.

Slowly lift your torso to a standing position, still holding your hands and arms behind you, to prepare for the Lateral Side Stretch and Full Length Stretch.

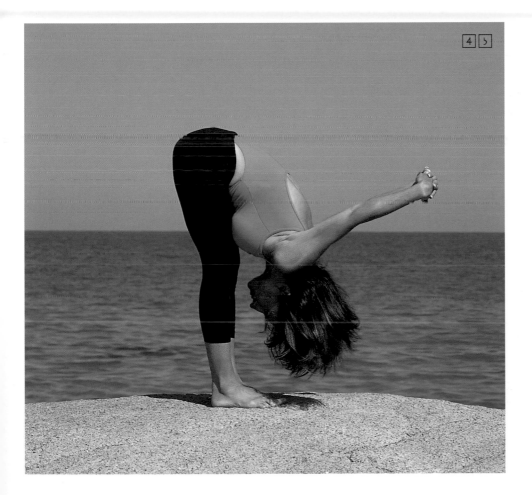

Lateral Side Stretch and
Full Length Stretch

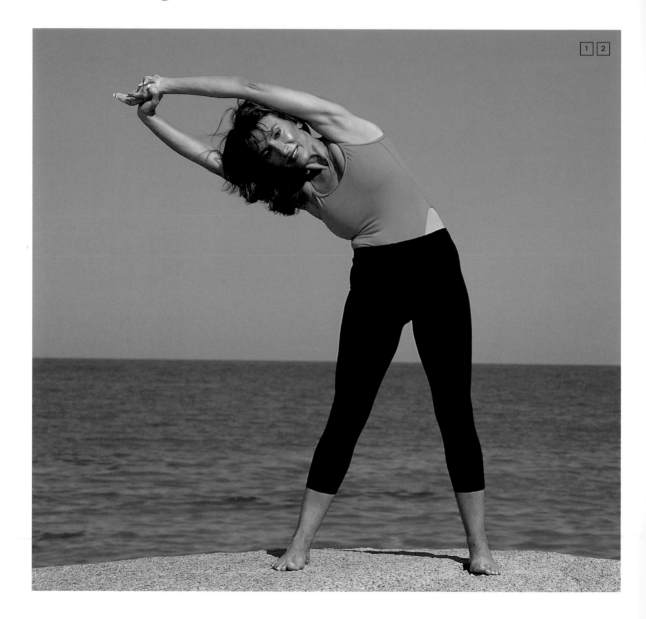

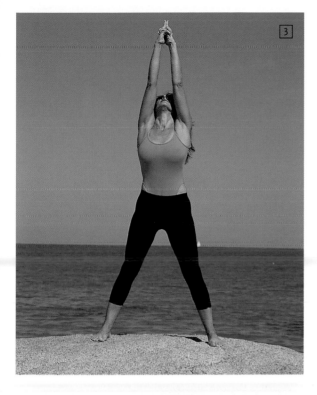

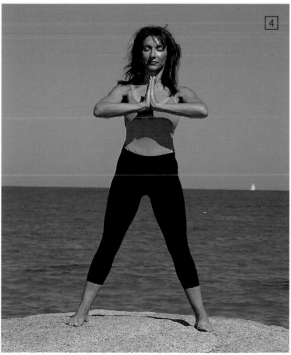

DIRECTIONS

1 Standing straight up, unclasp your hands and grab hold of your left wrist with your right hand. Stretch all the way over to the right.

2 Slowly return your body to standing straight, and switch hands, grabbing your right wrist with your left hand. Stretch all the way over to the left.

3 Slowly return your body to standing straight, release your hand, and interlace your fingers with your index fingers pointing upwards. Stretch your arms all the way over your head and gently release your head back. Feel the stretch from your waist all the way up to your pointed fingers.

4 Bring your hands to your heart center and close your eyes. Take 2 long, deep breaths, inhaling and exhaling completely, reaching down to the bottom part of your lungs.

Sun Salutation

Sun Salutations are made up of a series of poses, including standing poses, Plank, Chaturanga, Upward Facing Dog, and Downward Facing Dog. This series of poses awakens every inch of the body, imparting benefits to both the muscular and skeletal systems. Sun Salutations add suppleness to the spine, moving it in a backward and forward motion, and bring some flexibility to the shoulders, neck, arms, and hamstrings. They also jump-start the cardiovascular system through continuous movement of the body.

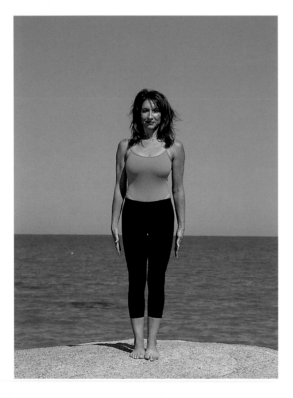
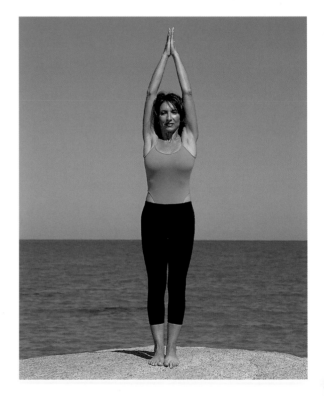

DIRECTIONS

1 Align your body, placing your feet together and your hands at your sides.

2 Inhale, roll your arms out with the palms facing out toward the ceiling, and bring your palms together overhead.

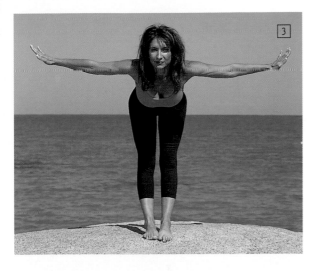

 3 Exhale, roll your arms out to the side and toward the floor, and gently release your head down toward the floor, lengthening your spine. Place your hands flat on the floor beside your feet.

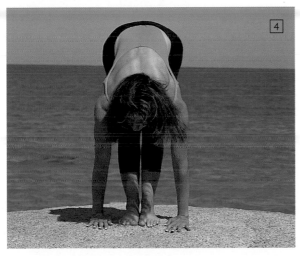

4 Inhale and lift your head up.

5 Exhale and release your head toward the floor.

Keep your hands on the floor and bring your right leg and then your left leg back, so your body is parallel to the floor and ready for Plank Pose.

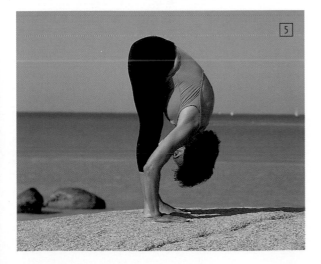

Plank Pose
(Sun Salutation, continued)

This is a weight-bearing pose. It will strengthen and prepare you for the other upper body poses that are more intense.

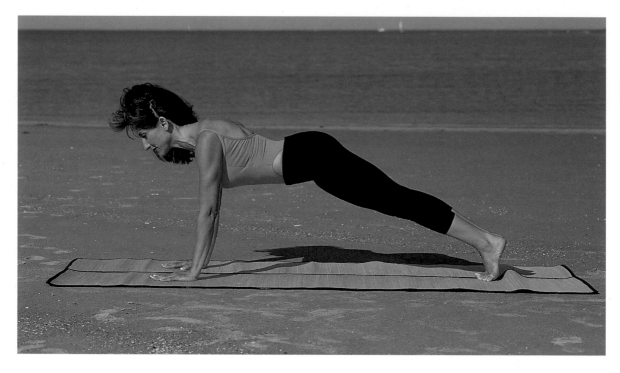

DIRECTIONS

1 Position your hands flat on the floor under your shoulders. Make sure they're pointing directly forward.

2 Tuck your toes under and come onto the balls of your feet, stretching through your heels.

3 Activate both thighs while keeping the back of your body really firm and flat.

4 Press firmly into your hands, and look toward the floor.

Continue directly into either the Modified Chaturanga or Challenge Chaturanga Pose.

Modified Chaturanga Pose
(Sun Salutation, continued)

Chaturanga is the Sanskrit term for a modified push-up. The pose will help you develop strength in your upper body and start to reshape your arms and shoulders.

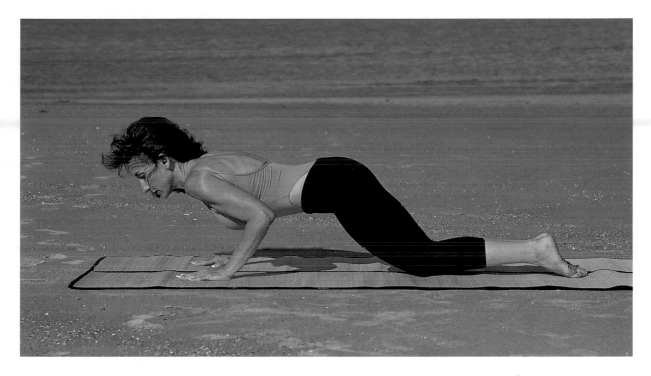

DIRECTIONS

1 Lower your knees to the floor, still keeping the muscles of your legs engaged.

2 Bend your elbows back, keeping them close to your body. Keep your shoulders square and gaze toward the floor.

3 Bend your elbows and bring your chest toward the floor, keeping your shoulders in line with your elbows, not lower, and keeping your body as straight as can be. Hold for 5 breaths.

Challenge Chaturanga Pose
(Sun Salutation, continued)

When you have sufficient strength, perform this pose in place of the Modified Chaturanga. This pose is used often, and needs special attention if you're going to master it.

DIRECTIONS

1 Remain in Plank Pose, with your knees off the floor.

2 Lower your upper body by bending your elbows, tucking them in, and hugging your ribcage. Continue to keep your body firm and supported; don't let it sag to the floor. If this happens, place your knees to the floor in Modified Chaturanga Pose.

3 Keep your elbows as close to your body as you can and your palms flat on the floor.

4 Lengthen your spine and keep your thighs active as you tighten your tummy muscles and gaze toward the floor. Hold the pose for 5 breaths.

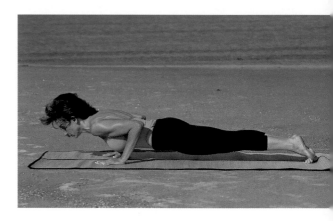

COMMON PROBLEMS

1. Hands aren't directly under your shoulders.
2. Elbows aren't tucked in.
3. Not enough strength for Challenge Chaturanga.
4. Looking up, rather than gazing toward the floor.
5. Leading with your nose, rather than your chest, as you lower yourself toward the floor.
6. Allowing your shoulder blades to "cave in" toward each other.

From the Modified or Challenge Chaturanga, continue directly into Upward Facing Dog.

Upward Facing Dog
(Sun Salutation, continued)

This pose really starts to warm up the spine with a gentle backbend. It will also open your chest and strengthen your arms and shoulders.

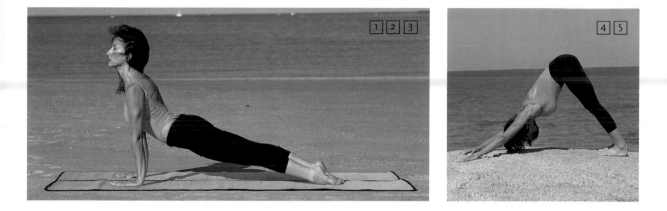

DIRECTIONS

1 From either Chaturanga Pose, scoop your chest and move your whole body forward and upward, rolling forward over the tops of your toes into Upward Facing Dog.

2 Open and lift your chest, straighten your arms, and lift your body so that only your hands and the tops of your feet support your body. Try and lift your thighs off the floor by tightening your thighs and buttocks.

3 Arch your spine and gaze directly in front of you, or gently drop your head back.

4 Curl your toes under, lift your hips, and stretch back into Downward Facing Dog.

5 Repeat the Sun Salutation series 2 or 3 times.

Full Locust Pose *(Backbend I)*

This pose gradually arches your back and is invaluable for strengthening your lower back muscles, an area that seldom gets any strength-building.

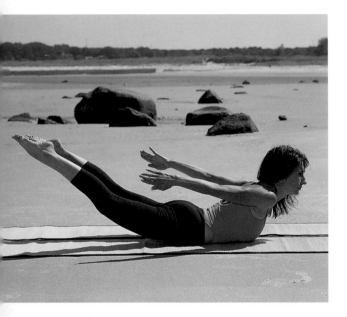

THE FULL-LOCUST POSE firms your back, buttocks, and hips, prevents back problems, and massages your internal organs, which results in improved functioning of the digestive system.

ANTIAGING TIP

This pose will help you develop

a youthful spine as your muscles and nerves

get stretched and strengthened.

DIRECTIONS

1 Lie flat on your stomach, and keep both your hips on the floor. Stretch your arms out alongside your body, and inhale.

2 Exhale, lifting your chest and thighs off the floor and your arms back and up, like wings. Keep your legs as straight as you can, extended back and up, and slightly apart. Lead with your chest, not your head, which should be in a neutral position.

3 Stretch through your arms and legs, and hold the pose for 5 breaths. Repeat the pose 3 times, slowly releasing your body to the floor at the end of the last repetition.

COMMON PROBLEMS

1. Neck strain; try to keep your head in a neutral position.
2. Overextending to the point of pain.

Spinal Extension *(Backbend II)*

In this pose, your arms are forward, your legs are stretched back, and you're lifting your opposite arm and leg to stretch and tone your back muscles.

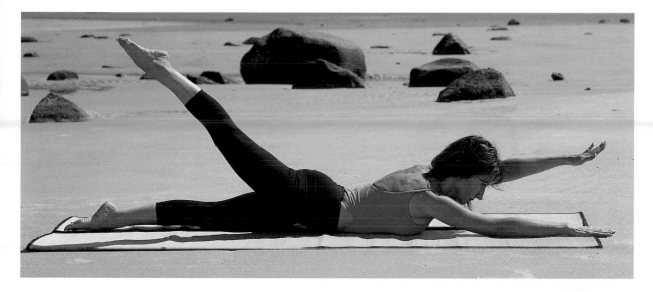

DIRECTIONS

1 Lie facedown on the floor, arms stretched out in front of you.

2 Inhale, lifting and extending your right arm forward and your left leg back and away from your body.

3 Exhale, and lift your raised limbs off the ground to a challenging height. Hold the pose for 5 breaths.

4 Lower your arm and leg to the ground, raise the opposite arm and leg, and repeat the pose.

THE SPINAL EXTENSION strengthens the backside of your body and creates a long curve of the spine.

COMMON PROBLEMS

1. Neck strain; try to keep your head in a neutral position.

2. Not lengthening and lifting for extension.

ANTIAGING TIP

This pose increases circulation to the spine and massages and stimulates the adrenal glands and kidneys for improved functioning.

Bow Pose *(Backbend III)*

This is an intense backbend that stretches your entire spine and all the muscles along it.

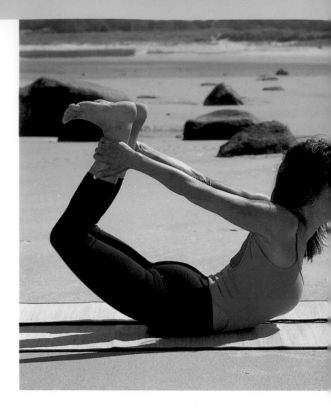

THE BOW POSE strengthens your spine and massages your back muscles.

DIRECTIONS

1. Lie flat on your stomach. Bend your knees, and move them about hip-width apart.

2. Reach backward with straight arms and grasp your ankles. Inhale.

3. Exhale, and as you arch your entire body upward, pull back with your legs, raising your head, chest, and thighs off the floor. Hold for 5 breaths.

4. Lower your body slowly to the ground. Repeat the pose twice.

ANTIAGING TIP

This pose will bring relief to tight, immovable muscles along the spine.

COMMON PROBLEMS

1. Improper hand placement; grab your ankles, not your feet.
2. Elbows are bent, instead of straight.
3. Knees are bent too sharply and the heels are down on the buttocks.
4. Only the upper body is lifted off the floor.
5. Knees wider than hip width apart.
6. Neck strain; try to keep your head in a neutral position.

✿ MODIFICATION

If you cannot reach your ankles with your hands, wrap a small towel or strap around each ankle and pull back with your legs and straight arms.

Child's Pose

Arms Stretched Forward

This is a very important counter pose to the backbends you just performed.

DIRECTIONS

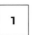 **1** Kneel on the floor and bring your buttocks toward your heels.

 2 Place your palms on the ground right in front of you, reaching forward with your arms.

3 Relax your neck muscles, bring your forehead to the floor, and relax into Child's Pose.

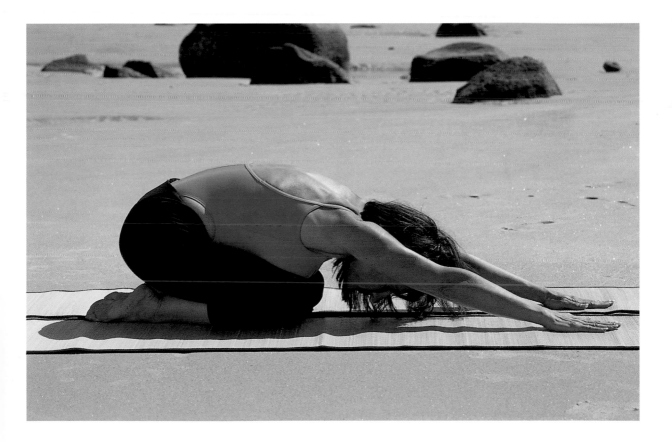

Bridge Pose

In this pose, your body takes the shape of a bridge. This pose will make your back and hips supple, and it's great for toning thigh and buttocks muscles.

DIRECTIONS

1 Lie flat on your back and bend your knees, placing the soles of your feet flat on the floor with your heels touching or close to your buttocks.

2 Turn your toes in slightly, making sure your feet and knees are slightly wider than hip-width apart.

3 Keep your arms down by your sides while you raise and squeeze your thighs and buttocks, arching your back upward. Lift your hips high, and raise your chest and navel as high as possible without moving your feet or shoulders. Your feet should remain flat on the floor.

4 Bring your arms under your body, interlace your fingers, and straighten your arms flat on the ground, pressing them into the floor. Hold the pose for 10 breaths.

CHALLENGE

Hold the pose for 20 breaths.

COMMON PROBLEMS

1. Hips and chest not arched up high enough.
2. Heels are raised off the floor. Feet should be flat on the floor, directly under the knees.
3. Feet and knees are turned out.
4. Shoulders or head lifted off the floor.

MODIFICATION

Listen to your body as you lift your hips as far as you comfortably can, and if you feel strain in your knees, just move your heels a little further away from your torso.

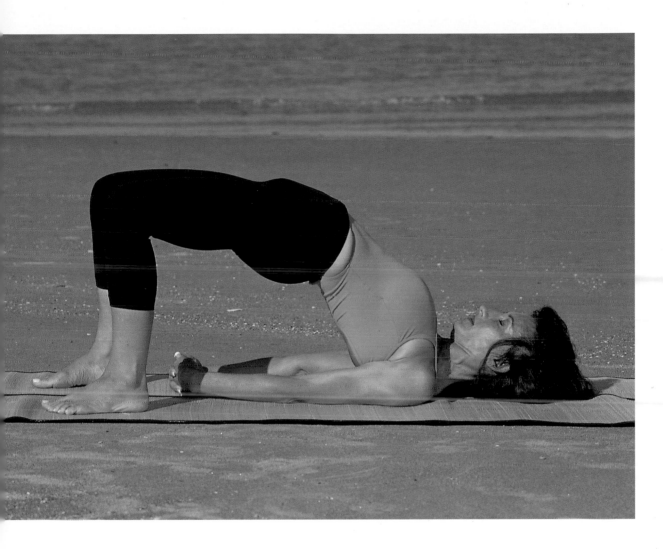

ANTIAGING TIP

The pose will make your spine, hips, and thighs more
youthful and will increase spine mobility. As you
contract your thighs and buttocks, you will contract
your pelvic floor, strengthening those muscles, too.

THE BRIDGE POSE firms your thighs and buttocks,
eliminates rounded shoulders, and realigns your spine,
which relieves backache.

Seated Forward Bend

The Seated Forward Bend gives an intense stretch to the back of the body as you fold forward.

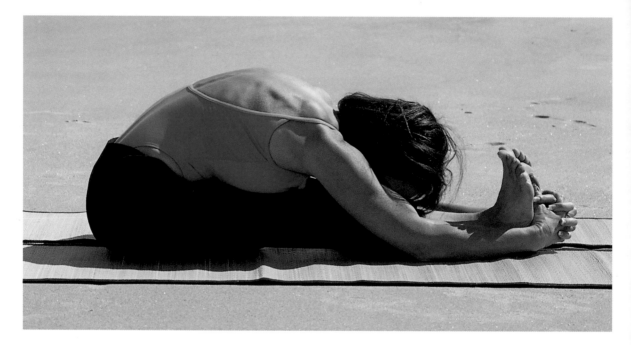

DIRECTIONS

1 Sit with your legs stretched out in front of you, knees straight. Pull your toes back toward your body.

2 Lift your arms, elongating your spine and stretching your entire back up and forward.

3 Hinge at the hips and fall forward, grabbing your feet or wherever you can reach, whether it's your toes, heels, ankles, or shins. Bring your chest down toward your thighs, never forcing the stretch.

4 Relax your shoulders and your neck, and look toward your legs. Hold the pose for 5 breaths.

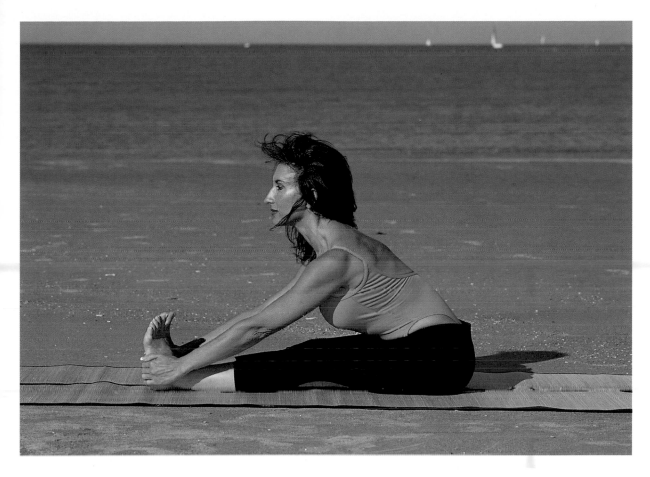

COMMON PROBLEMS

1. Rounding your back and bringing your head toward your knees, rather than your chest and chin toward your legs.
2. Not hinging from the waist. You need to work through extending your spine.
3. Allowing the feet to come apart or flop open to the sides.
4. Forgetting to pull your toes back.

ANTIAGING TIP

In this pose you're not only getting the benefits of an intense stretch to the backside of the body, you're also massaging your abdominal organs for better digestion.

THE SEATED FORWARD BEND stretches your lower back and hamstrings, and relieves compression of your spine.

🌸 MODIFICATION

Tight hips? Modify this pose by placing a rolled towel under your sitting bones. This will allow you to fold forward a lot easier without straining your lower back. Also try bending your knees and easing forward from your hips, or using a small towel or strap around your feet.

Inclined Plane Pose

A counter pose, the Inclined Plane complements the complete stretch given to the back of the body in the Seated Forward Bend. You hold your body in a reverse plank position, facing upwards.

DIRECTIONS

1. Sit with your legs stretched forward.

2. Place the palms of your hands on the floor on either side of your body, just behind your buttocks, fingers facing forward.

3. Raise your buttocks and lift your body upward, pushing your hips up and making your body as straight and as much like a plank as possible.

4. Let your head hang back and down gently, and keep the soles of your feet flat on the ground and your arms and legs straight. Hold the pose for 5 breaths.

MODIFICATION

Be very cautious with this pose if you have a neck problem. If the pose really bothers you, keep your chin up and look forward, or keep your head in a neutral position.

COMMON PROBLEMS

1. Letting your feet fall open and to the side, instead of keeping them together.
2. Tensing your neck and shoulders.
3. Placing your hands out of line with your shoulders.

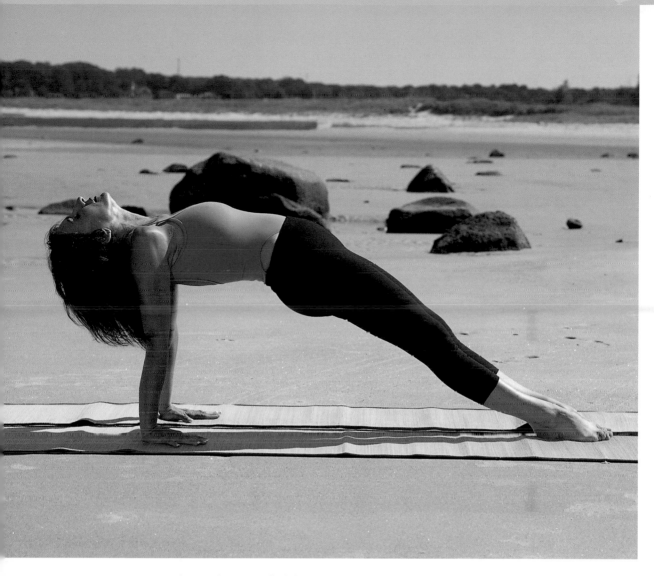

THE INCLINED PLANE POSE strengthens and increases flexibility in your shoulders, arms, and hips, and tones the lumbar region of your spine and your Achilles.

ANTIAGING TIP

This is an empowering posture—and very rejuvenating—because you use every muscle, tendon, and ligament in your body to hold yourself in the pose. It's strengthening for the whole body.

Abdominal I

This pose isolates and works the entire abdomen. Proper technique is very important throughout the abdominal exercises, because if the stomach muscles are not strong enough to perform the exercise properly, other muscles will compensate, which could lead to injury. Your abdominal muscles are the most important muscles in your body. They're your center, the core from which all movement radiates. This physical core provides the foundation for good posture and strength. Strong abdominal muscles will take the pressure off your lower back.

DIRECTIONS

1. Lie flat on the floor with your knees bent. Interlace your hands behind the base of your head, keeping your elbows open to support your neck as you raise your head off the floor. (This works upper abdominal muscles.)

2. Pull your abdominal muscles into your back as you bring your knees toward your chest. This is the most vital part of performing this exercise correctly. Extend your knees slightly, to work your lower abdominal muscles.

3. Inhale, and as you pull your abdominals toward your back, consciously feel your back flatten into the floor. If at any moment you arch your spine, you immediately put stress on your lower back and you do not get the maximum benefit of this exercise. It is vital that you maintain a flat back throughout this exercise.

4. Exhale, keep your back flat on the floor, and lift your shoulder blades off the floor as you crunch, working the entire abdominal region. The range of movement is small, and you should move slowly.

5. Lift and lower your shoulder blades 10 to 20 times. Release your abdominals and bring both your knees in toward your chest.

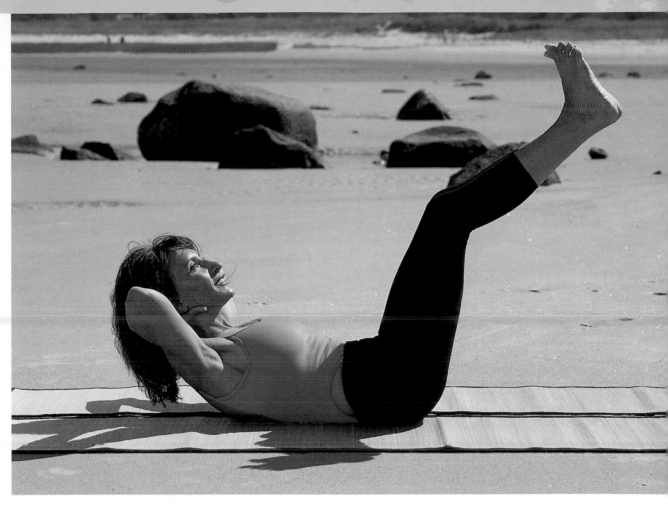

THE ABDOMINAL EXERCISE POSE tones your stomach muscles and slims your waistline, as well as strengthen the spine for better posture.

COMMON PROBLEMS

1. Straining the neck by not maintaining correct alignment of the head and neck.
2. Allowing the back to lift off the floor, using the lower back muscles.

CHALLENGE

Try to complete 3 sets of 20.

ANTIAGING TIP

Did you know that weak abdominal muscles can actually cause back problems to occur? If your stomach muscles are weak, your posture is most likely off, and that makes it easier for vertebrae to slip out of alignment. Simple back movements can then result in pulled back muscles. How aging is that?

Abdominal II

This pose activates the upper and lower abs to develop a firm center.

DIRECTIONS

1 Lie on your back with your knees bent. Interlace your hands behind your neck, placing your thumbs on either side of your neck.

2 Inhale and lift your head off the floor, supporting your head with your hands and keeping your elbows out to the sides. Lift your shoulders off the floor to engage your abdominal muscles.

3 Tighten and pull in your lower abdominals as you lift your legs in a bent position.

4 Exhale and lower your right leg toward the floor. Flex your foot, keep your spine absolutely flat on the floor, and make sure your abs are not bulging out as you lower your leg as far as you can while maintaining proper positioning.

5 Repeat 10 times with each leg, alternating sides. Release your abs and bring your knees into your chest.

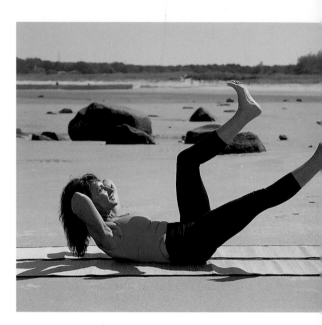

CHALLENGE

Try to do 3 sets of Abdominal II.

COMMON PROBLEMS

1. Letting your abs bulge out as you lower your leg toward the floor.

2. Lowering your legs too far toward the floor, causing your spine to arch. This will cause lower back strain.

Abdominal III

This is the perfect pose to shape and contour your waist.

DIRECTIONS

1 Lie on your back with your knees bent. Interlace your hands behind your neck, placing your thumbs on either side of your neck to support your head.

2 Inhale, and lift your head and shoulder blades off the floor, keeping your elbows out to the sides and supporting your head to engage your upper abs.

3 Tighten and pull in your lower abs as you lift your legs, bent at a 90-degree angle.

4 Exhale, keeping your back flat on the floor, and extend your left leg out as you bring your left elbow toward your right knee. Remember to keep your elbows open and your lower abdominals pulled in toward your back tight.

5 Inhale, change legs, and exhale to the other side. This exercise is done at a brisker pace and will engage the obliques. Repeat 10 to 20 times per side.

Release your abs and bend both knees into your chest for Knees to Chest Pose.

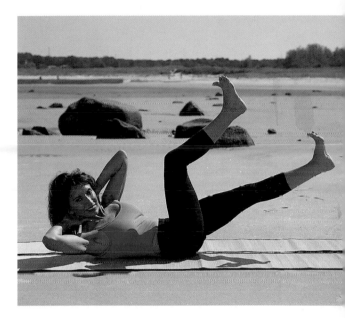

CHALLENGE

Perform 3 sets of this exercise.

Knees to Chest Pose

This pose will immediately release your abdominals as your press your spine flat into the floor.

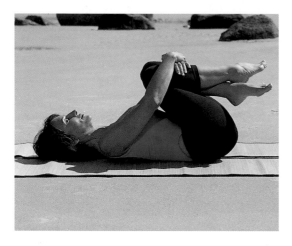

THE KNEES TO CHEST POSE releases your abdominals and stretches your lower back.

DIRECTIONS

 1 Bring both knees in tight to your chest.

2 Wrap both arms around your knees in a hug, and hold for a few breaths, or until you feel your spine and abs relax.

Spinal Balancing and Hip Rotation

The first part of this exercise improves balance and lengthens your spine as you stretch from your fingertips to your toes. In the second part, as you bring your leg out to the side, you open your hips and pelvis for improved flexibility as you tone those thigh and buttocks muscles.

DIRECTIONS

1 Begin the pose on all fours, knees under your hips, hands under your shoulders.

 2 Extend your right arm forward and your left leg back, holding them parallel to the floor. Stretch your spine from your fingertips to your toes, using all your strength. Feel the energy extend from the center of your body in both directions.

 3 Gaze down at the floor, being careful not to lift your head. Hold the pose for 5 breaths.

ANTIAGING TIP

This is a wonderful posture for achieving maximum flexibility in your hips, where most of us are completely rigid and stiff at any age.

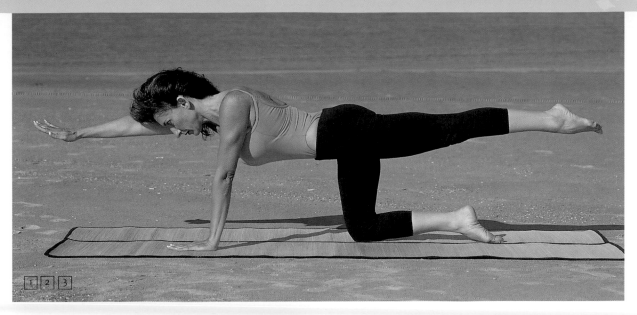

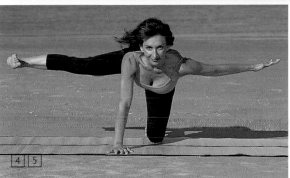

THE SPINAL BALANCING AND HIP ROTATION POSE tones your thighs, buttocks, arms, and back, as well as lengthen your spine, engage your abdominals, and flex your hips.

4 Extend your right arm out to the side at shoulder level and your left leg out to the side at hip level. Hold this pose for 10 breaths.

5 Repeat one more time with the same arm and leg, and then repeat with the opposite arm and leg.

MODIFICATION

If you have knee problems, double up your mat and place a towel under each knee. Practice this pose to your own degree; as your hips get more flexible, your leg will be able to extend a little further out to the side.

COMMON PROBLEMS

1. Lifting your head and throwing your spine out of alignment; especially in spinal extension, your head should face down toward the floor.
2. Placing your hands incorrectly; they should be under your shoulders.
3. Letting your hips twist to one side, rather than squaring them forward during the spinal extension, or not opening the hips as you bring your leg out to the side.

CHALLENGE

Try to perform 2 sets of 10 on each side.

Child's Pose

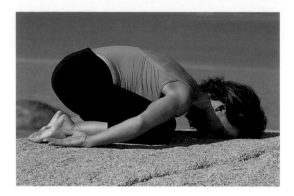

DIRECTIONS

1	Kneel on the floor and bring your buttocks toward your heels.
2	Place your arms lengthwise, alongside your body.
3	Stretch your chin forward and gently lower your forehead to the floor, rounding your spine and shoulders.
4	Relax your neck muscles and relax into the pose.

Remain in Child's Pose for Dolphin with Leg and Buttocks Toning Pose.

MODIFIED POSE

If your forehead does not touch the floor when your buttocks are close to your heels, open your knees slightly, allowing your forehead to touch the floor. Place a pillow under your head, if necessary, until you gain the necessary flexibility.

Dolphin with Leg and Buttocks Toning Pose

This pose will build tremendous upper-body strength and tone your arms and shoulders while simultaneously toning and reshaping your thighs and buttocks.

DIRECTIONS

1	From Child's Pose, place your elbows on the floor in front of you, interlace your fingers, and lift your head off the floor. Continue looking toward the floor, keeping your head in a neutral position.
2	Straighten your legs, lifting your hips and squaring them forward.
3	Lift your right leg straight behind you, flex your foot, and activate every muscle in your leg as you squeeze and tighten your buttocks.
4	Lift and lower your leg 5 times.
5	Bring your knees back to the floor, and perform 5 repetitions with the other leg.

CHALLENGE

Work up to 10 repetitions per side.

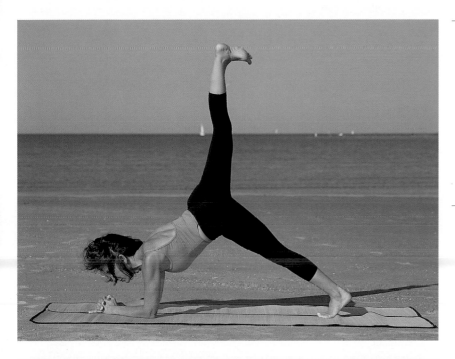

ANTIAGING TIP

By toning, reshaping, and strengthening your whole body, this pose will refresh your whole system. Plus, the inversion brings blood to your head, reversing the effects of gravity.

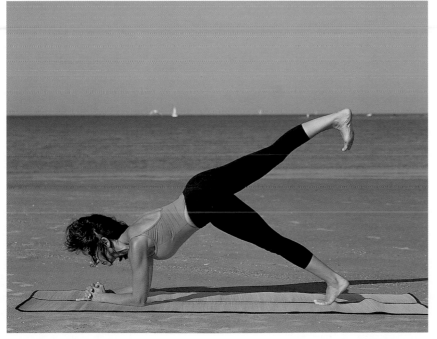

Shoulder and Arm Stretch

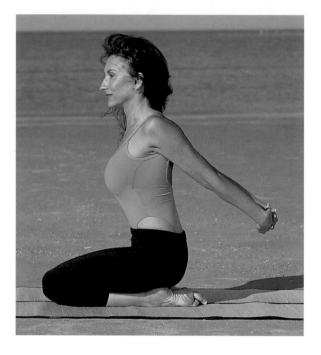

Runner's Lunge Pose

This is a full hip abductor stretch, stretching and lengthening the hip muscles and rotator muscles of the buttocks.

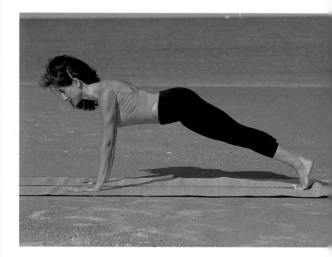

DIRECTIONS

1	Kneel on the floor with your spine straight, and interlace your hands behind your back.
2	With your shoulders back and your arms straight, lift your arms as high as you can, feeling a good stretch in your arms and shoulders. Hold the pose for a few breaths.

1	Get into Plank Position by placing your hands on the floor directly under your shoulders. Make sure your fingers are pointing forward. Extend your legs with your toes tucked under, and hold your body so your back is flat.

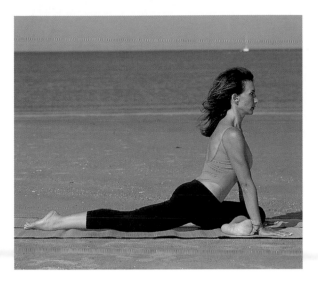

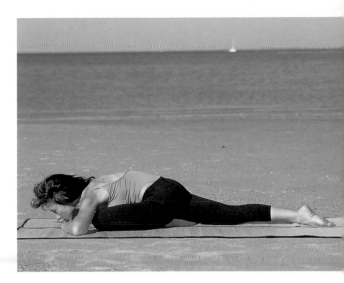

THE RUNNER'S LUNGE POSE opens and stretches your external hip rotator muscles and works the psoas muscle and the groin of your back leg.

2 Bring your left leg forward under your body, at a 90-degree angle or less, depending on the flexibility of your hips and any knee problems you might have.

3 Slowly drop your bent knee to the floor and lower your body down over the bent leg. Your body should be straight and squared forward, not twisted, and your back leg should extend straight behind you.

4 Inhale, extend your chest up, and exhale, sinking your chest toward the floor.

5 Bring your arms forward and hold the pose for 5 breaths.

6 Switch legs and repeat the pose.

CHALLENGE

Hold the pose for 10 breaths.

 MODIFICATION

If you have had knee surgery or suffer from knee pain, be cautious with this pose, or perform the Hip Rotation Pose (see page 164) in its place.

Open Angle Pose

You'll reap tremendous benefits from the intense hamstring stretch this pose provides. You'll also stretch your inner legs and open your hips and groin. And as you stretch forward and then to the sides, you'll gain flexibility in your spine.

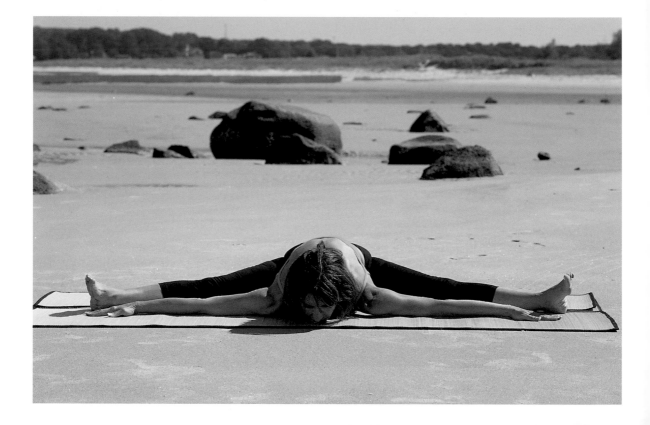

DIRECTIONS

1 Spread your legs wide apart and press your hamstrings and calf muscles to the floor. Flex your feet and sit tall.

2 Stretch your arms over your head, lengthening your spine, and bend from the waist. When your hands touch the ground, gently walk them forward until you feel a good stretch. Ultimately you want to reach final position, where your chest and chin rest on the floor and your arms are extended all the way to each side.

3 Make sure your spine stays long and extended, and be conscious of releasing your neck muscles. Hold the pose for 5 breaths.

4 For an extra stretch, crawl your torso toward your right leg and walk your hands as far forward as you can, reaching for your right foot. Hold the pose for 5 breaths, then repeat with your left leg.

Return to the pose's starting position and prepare for the Lateral Torso Stretch.

CHALLENGE

Hold the pose for 10 breaths.

🌸 MODIFICATION

Sit on the edge of a folded blanket and wrap a towel or strap around each leg. Hold them there with your arms extended, and tilt your pelvis forward, being careful not to round your back.

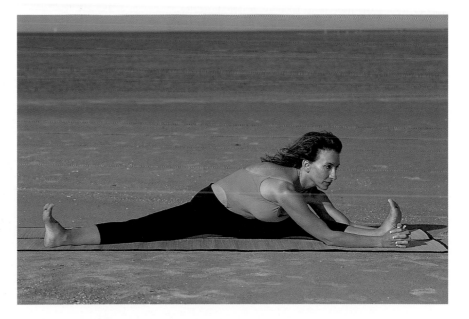

Lateral Torso Stretch

This pose starts in the same position as Open Angle Pose, but extends your body all the way to each side, giving your waist and spine a good, strong stretch.

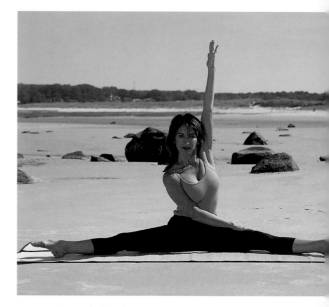

DIRECTIONS

1 With your legs spread wide and your hamstring and calf muscles pressed to the floor, grab your left thigh with your right hand and extend your left arm toward the ceiling.

2 Bring your right shoulder toward your right thigh, leaning over to get a wonderful stretch to the side of the waist. Hold for 5 breaths.

3 Repeat the pose to the other side.

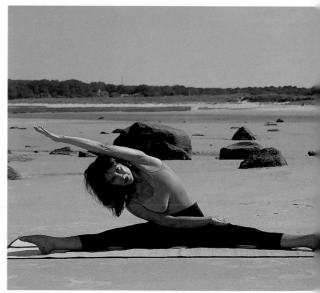

Lying Down Spinal Twist

This twist is relaxing and easy to practice. It's simple and gentle, yet entirely stretches the muscles in your back and hips. This posture is wonderful to use near the end of the routine to release the muscles in your lower back.

DIRECTIONS

1. Lie flat on the floor, arms stretched out to the side and palms pressing into the floor.

2. Inhale, bend your left leg and wrap your right thigh over your left thigh, entwining your legs and keeping your back on the floor.

3. Exhale and bring your legs over to the left, twisting your spine to the right as you turn your head to the right.

4. Slowly bring your legs back to the center, uncross and recross your legs the opposite way, and repeat the pose to the opposite side.

ANTIAGING TIP

Whether you are very active or more sedentary, everyday life causes a lot of abuse to the spine. This gentle twist helps your spine recuperate.

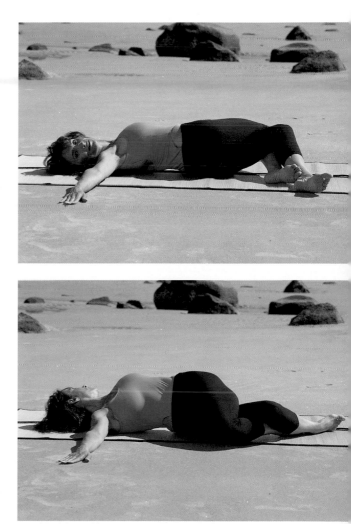

Plough Pose

Plough is an inverted pose. The forward bending action will massage and stimulate your thyroid gland, and as you roll forward you will feel the stretching in your shoulders and neck.

A Note on Plough into Shoulder Stand:

These postures have many, many benefits, but they're not recommended for anyone who has high blood pressure, a heart condition (including hypertension), or eye problems (including glaucoma). If you do not fall into these categories of illness, you can put these poses into your routine. Alternatively, you can use the Legs Against the Wall inverted posture just before Savasana.

DIRECTIONS

1 Lie on your back with your head and neck straight, looking up toward the ceiling.

2 With your arms on the floor and palms down for support, gently lift your knees to your chest. Keeping your knees bent, lift your buttocks and roll your legs over your head, straightening your legs until your toes are touching the floor.

3 Bring the palms of your hands to your lower back and hold the pose for 5 breaths, breathing normally.

MODIFICATION

If you can't quite touch the floor with your toes, let them just point behind you above the floor behind your head. With practice, your toes will reach the ground.

COMMON PROBLEMS

1. Legs are not straight in full plow.

2. Head and neck are twisted to one side.

3. Back is arched, rather than flat.

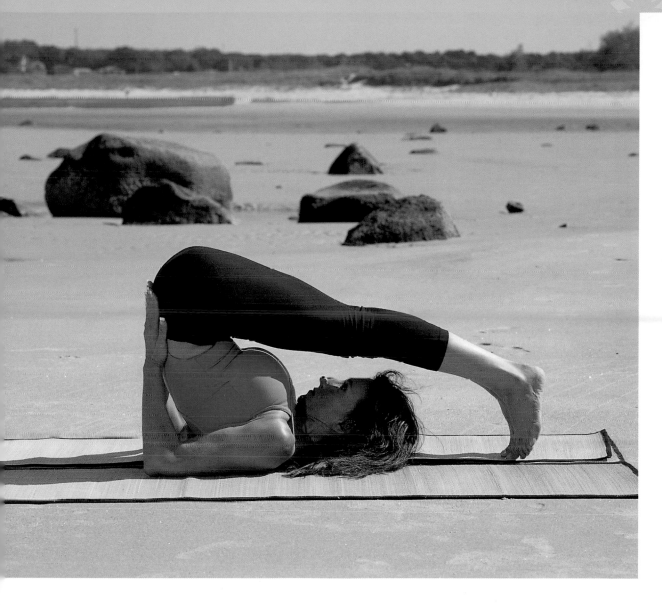

This forward bending action and inversion
will stimulate the sex glands and increase
flexibility of the spine—a great combination
for increasing libido.

THE PLOUGH POSE relieves stiffness in your shoulders and neck,
increases spinal flexibility, and stimulates your thyroid glands,
liver, kidneys, and spleen.

Shoulder Stand

This inverted pose is called the "Queen of postures" because of its therapeutic qualities. In this pose, you support your body with your hands and elbows and balance on your shoulders.

DIRECTIONS

1. While in Plough Pose, walk your hands to your spine, making sure your elbows are evenly positioned.

2. Straighten your back as much as possible and raise your legs perpendicular to the floor, supporting your back on your elbows. Hold the pose for 5 breaths, breathing normally.

3. Come out of the position by lowering your feet to a 45-degree angle over your head, and move back into Plough before you slowly lower your body back onto the floor, one vertebra at a time. Bend your knees if necessary as you gradually unroll your body and relax into Savasana.

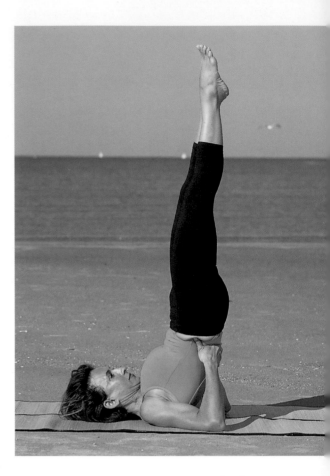

THE SHOULDER STAND POSE reverses gravity, thereby alleviating the appearance of varicose veins, stimulating your thyroid and endocrine glands, and reinvigorating internal organs.

COMMON PROBLEMS

1. Elbows are placed too far apart.
2. Head and neck are twisted to one side.
3. Breathing is erratic or held while in the pose.
4. Legs are not together.

ANTIAGING TIP

This inverted posture reverses the effects of gravity—meaning your heart and brain receive a healthy rush of blood—and when you come out of the pose you will feel refreshed and rejuvenated. Inversion poses have very strong positive effects on the entire body.

Legs Against the Wall

Relaxing with your legs up against a wall is also an inversion, and it's a great alternative if you need to modify Shoulder Stand. There are many great benefits of this simple inverted pose, especially for people who stand for long periods of time, or who have varicose veins and swollen, red feet.

Perform this modification as necessary, and as soon as health conditions improve, graduate to Shoulder Stand.

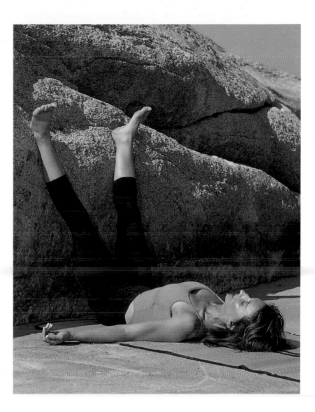

THE LEGS AGAINST THE WALL POSE increases circulation, and reverses the influence of gravity on your legs and internal organs.

DIRECTIONS

1 Get your buttocks as close to the wall as feels comfortable to you, straightening your legs up against the wall.

2 Place your legs a little more than hip width apart, and relax your legs.

3 Relax your head and your neck, and hold the pose for 10 breaths or longer. If you wish, you may stay in this position for Savasana.

ANTIAGING TIP

This is a great restorative yoga pose. By reversing gravity, the venous blood that would normally pool in the legs is easily returned to the heart, reducing the constriction of arteries throughout the body.

Savasana, or Corpse Pose

DIRECTIONS

 1 Lie flat on your back with your feet apart and your toes relaxed and facing out.

2 Place your arms slightly out from your sides, with your palms up.

3 Close your eyes and consciously release and relax each and every muscle, transferring all the weight of your body to the floor.

4 Slowly bring your focus to your breath, and feel the rhythmic movement of your body as you breathe in and out. Really get in touch with your body and your breath, holding the pose for 5 to 10 minutes.

5 Wrap your arms around your knees, drawing them into your chest, and roll to your right side into a fetal position.

From this position, roll onto your knees to prepare for Child's Pose.

✿ MODIFICATION

If your lower back feels uncomfortable lying in Savasana, bend your knees instead of straightening your legs.

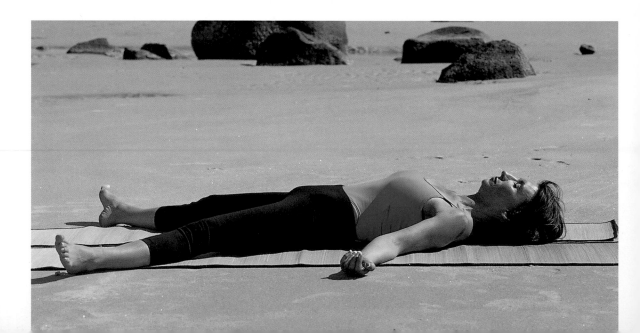

Child's Pose

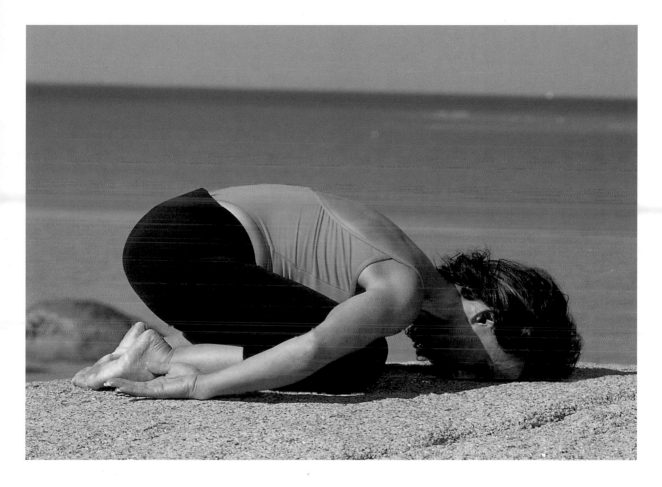

DIRECTIONS

 1 Kneel on the floor and bring your buttocks toward your heels.

 2 Place your arms lengthwise, alongside your body.

3 Stretch your chin forward and gently lower your forehead to the floor, rounding your spine and shoulders.

4 Relax your neck muscles and relax into the pose. Hold the pose for 3 breaths.

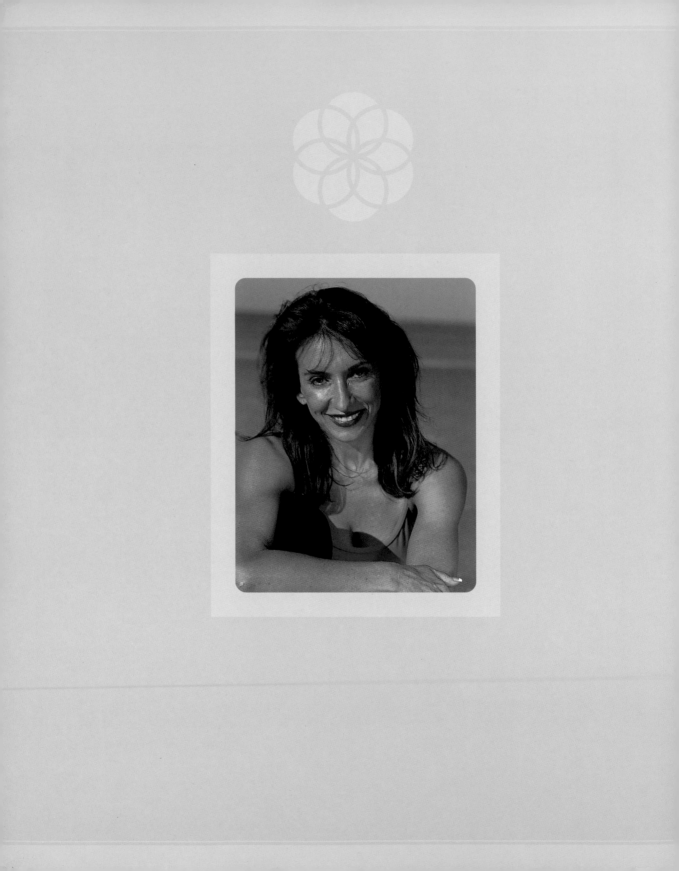

Chapter 6

Staying Motivated

In the end, the body's most powerful muscle is the mind. Remember that this program is a process. The first time you practice the routines, it will be extremely elemental and awkward. Don't let that stop you. Be gentle and positive with yourself. You'll improve. The second time you practice, the routine will get easier, and the following time will be even easier than that.

I always tell my students about the "Magic Three," meaning it usually requires three sessions before the magic of movement begins. In most cases, students will really start getting a feel for the program after the first three sessions. At this point, something "kicks in," and the repetition of the postures and routines begins to guide you. That locomotion in itself will be a motivation as you start to feel and see the changes yoga produces.

And always remember: You don't have to be a yoga master to gain the tremendous antiaging benefits of yoga. Most of the benefits come from simple, basic postures, as shown in this book, practiced to whatever degree the practitioner is comfortable with. Yoga postures can look very beautiful and graceful in photos, but keep in mind that the most important part is not how you look, but how your body is benefiting. It's all about growth: building your strength, your flexibility, and your state of mind. Eventually the poses do become more graceful and easier to achieve, but don't worry about that until you get there.

Even with the most successful routines, though, there will be the occasional temptation to skip practice because something else seems to need your immediate attention. Here are a few tips to staying motivated:

1   *Maintain a regular practice schedule, no matter what. We all know that "life" happens and there's always an excuse to put practice off for another day. But if you stay true to the time you've allotted to your yoga practice, you will see results, and that in itself will keep you motivated.*

2   *Calm your mind, listen to your body, and enjoy each pose. To do this, pace yourself and modify the poses, if necessary. Take longer in getting into a pose, if that works for you. Relax into the poses. This is not a marathon; it's a slow and gradual journey.*

3   *Always maintain a very relaxed and peaceful approach to your practice. Play music. Be joyful.*

4   *Respect your body, your limits, your strength, and your flexibility. Know that you'll get there when your body takes you there.*

5   *Gradually challenge yourself whenever you feel ready. Increase your workout and intensity at a pace that is good for you.*

Yoga is not a fad. It's a practice that can run through an entire lifetime. There are many exercises that pump up your body, but few programs that both feed your body and nourish your mind. As you go through this program, you'll experience firsthand that strong mind-body connection, and you'll see how powerful that connection can become. You will be encouraged and motivated as you gain awareness of how your body and mind work together to give you more clarity, stability, and confidence in every task you undertake and in everything you do.

MEDITATION

Meditation is at the heart of every style of yoga. Through meditation, yoga affects not only the body, but also the mind. Through meditation, you will experience peace, calm, and a greater sense of focus. There are many ways to meditate during this program.

Many of my students find that they are able to meditate much easier in their postures when they are moving; they find it easier than sitting still and trying to erase thoughts from their minds. So try it. You may need to try several different approaches during your yoga session before you discover what works best for you and pursue that approach.

Once your yoga advances through the program, yoga will become a meditation in itself. I have become so focused, so in the moment, that I meditate not only throughout my personal sessions, but also throughout my busy classes. This ability came with time. You can meditate when you are walking or jogging, lying down or sitting. Narrowing the gaps between your thoughts and stilling your mind is the essence of meditation.

Yoga opens the hidden treasures of the mind and allows us to reap the incredible richness therein. We embrace the stillness, the openness, and the clarity of our world, which all too often get lost in the hustle of everyday living. By getting in touch with your core, your breath, and by staying in the moment in the postures, you will begin to meditate. This will happen subtly, as you progress. Be aware that it's happening and enjoy it for the wonder that it will bring to your life.

FOCUS ON YOUR BREATH

From the beginning, focus or concentrate on your breath, because the breath is the essence of meditation. A useful technique is to count your breaths during each pose, counting forward and backward, focusing your attention on what you are doing. Slow your breath with deep, long inhalations and exhalations. Stay with this technique throughout your session. This is the essence of meditation on breath.

FOCUS ON YOUR POSTURES

You can meditate during your practice by placing your total focus on the posture you are performing. Get in the moment and stay there. Focus on where you're placing your hand, your foot. Pay attention to how it feels to twist your spine, and feel your body's reaction to the challenging postures and stretches. Focus all your attention on what you are doing. This is meditation in motion.

FOCUS ON GAZING AT AN IMAGE

A successful portal into meditation is to gaze at an image during your yoga session. Think of something blissful and keep focusing on it in your mind. Whether it's a candle's flame or a loved one's face, keep it in the front of your mind and bring your attention back to it as you come into and go out of poses. You can also focus on something tangible in the room: a spot on the floor, something on the wall. It's amazing how focusing on a tangible object brings balance to both the body and mind. It's proof that the eye, and therefore the mind, controls the body.

FOCUS ON VISUALIZATION

Meditate during your session by visualizing yourself on a beautiful beach or in another natural place, experiencing the waves of the ocean, looking at the blue sky, hearing the sounds of nature. A CD of appropriate music can help you focus on your vision. It will give your mind a focal point and help you to still the chatter in your head.

ANTIAGING BENEFITS OF MEDITATION

As if the psychological benefits of meditation were not enough, there are clearly antiaging benefits to be gained from meditation, as well. With regular practice, you will find that meditation:

1. *Slows down brain activity and brings clarity.*

2. *Slows your rate of respiration and deepens breathing.*

3. *Decreases blood pressure.*

4. *Decreases mental stress and body tension.*

5. *Improves the quality of sleep; in most cases, you'll find less sleep is required.*

6. *Leaves you feeling refreshed, rejuvenated, and optimistic.*

Enjoy the Journey

You have started down the path toward eternal youth, for both your body and your mind. Do not look for instant gratification, but instead think of this as a journey that you have just begun. I can promise you that this yoga practice is a powerhouse and will deliver astounding results in stopping, then reversing, the aging process.

As you progress in your abilities, week after week, month after month, year after year, keep the following key points in mind. (You may want to refer back to this list if your progress plateaus, or just as a refresher from time to time.)

1. MOVE. *The program is composed of postures used in conjunction with Sun Salutations to create a cardiovascular effect that will rev up the metabolism for weight loss. This happens through constant movement, which is the "gas" that pushes this program to the level where the antiaging process begins. So keep moving. Shorten the gaps between postures, and you'll be amazed at the results.*

2. STRETCH. *Remember to include each of the stretches in between the postures. These stretches are the essence of youth. As you tighten your muscles for strength building, you must also lengthen them for flexibility, achieving a balanced approach to fitness.*

3. CONCENTRATE ON YOUR SPINE. *Of all of your body's bones and muscles, it is mostly your spine that dictates how you age. As you go from one posture to another, you'll move your spine in every direction, helping you achieve full flexibility for a young and supple spine. Opening the spaces between the vertebrae and lengthening the spine with the stretches will also help you avoid degeneration of the spine.*

4. FOCUS. *The balancing postures are designed to connect your mind and body, helping you achieve greater focus. You'll find that this will cross over into other areas of your life, giving you a greater and more focused attention span whatever your age. Bringing focus and deeper concentration is antiaging because it keeps the brain alert.*

5. USE YOUR OWN WEIGHT. *You will achieve a toned and sculptured body by strengthening your muscles in every pose. This is resistance training, using your body's own weight as a counterbalance in the strength-building poses. This builds bone mass and prevents or helps reverse the disabling effects of osteoporosis.*

6. STAY CALM. *You will achieve an inner calm and peace through practicing the postures. You will experience a genuine sense of outward tranquility, which transcends into a deeper state of inner peace. This will have a quieting and calming effect, reducing anxiety and agitation and helping you create a better, deeper, and more productive life.*

7. MEDITATE. *By meditating, you'll ensure that you will not only achieve a balanced and youthful figure, but also self-awareness and clarity. The total program will enhance your physical and mental health for a healthy young body and mind. So count your breath, focus on your postures, and learn how to meditate throughout the routines.*

8. WATCH YOUR DIET. *You will achieve a healthier body by fueling it with the highest quality food. See "Nutrition," below, to learn what changes you can make to help push yourself toward your goals. For some people, this may mean reducing coffee intake by a cup a day, or using olive oil instead of butter when cooking. Whatever small changes you make, you'll be taking an important step toward a younger you.*

NUTRITION

A healthy diet is absolutely mandatory if you want to stop and then reverse your body clock. Everything you eat becomes part of your body, your blood, your propensity to age. Food is digested into your bloodstream, and blood is transferred to every part of your body, either furnishing it with nourishment for building and maintaining optimum health or working against all your other efforts to improve your health. A poor diet is an invitation to aging. Not only does it lead to fatigue and stress, it slowly breaks the body down. Whether you are 16 or 60, a balanced dietary program, combined with the effects of yoga, will stop and then turn back the aging clock.

ANTIAGING DIET SUGGESTIONS

If you are already following some of these guidelines, good for you. If not, I suggest you choose one or two that seem like easy changes to incorporate—such as eating breakfast if you currently don't, or having a handful of nuts during the day—and add it to your routine. When that has become second nature to you, whether it's a few days or a few weeks from now, add another change or two. As your health improves, you'll stop thinking of them as changes and start thinking of them as permanent improvements to your life.

1. *Eat at regular intervals, never going more than five hours during the day without eating something, and don't skip breakfast. Your metabolism will slow down to compensate for the lack of food in your system, and that works against everything you're trying to achieve with this program.*

2. *Start to include lots of vegetables and fruits in your diet—aim for a minimum of five a day. These are loaded with vitamins, minerals, fiber, antioxidants, and phytonutrients.*

3. *Make sure you get your protein, but decrease the amount of meat and chicken in your diet and increase your consumption of fish, legumes, tofu, egg whites, and nuts. A handful of almonds make a choice snack.*

4. *Eliminate or decrease how much sugar, white flour, white rice, white potatoes, and fried food you eat.*

5. *Minimize your caffeine and alcohol intake, including wine.*

6. *Add oatmeal and brown rice to your diet, to make sure you're getting enough fiber.*

7. *Take vitamin and mineral supplements and omega-3 fatty acids for added support.*

Keep it simple and make some appropriate changes, and you'll be taking a giant step toward feeling and functioning better daily. Combine this with yoga, and you have the whole antiaging package.

PARTING THOUGHTS

Whenever beginning anything, whether it's a road trip or an exercise discipline, I always recall the great Deepak Chopra's famous comment, "Enjoy the journey, not the destination."

The journey is how we spend our lives. Rushing it works against us. The journey is the hour-by-hour, day-by-day, week-by-week process. The journey is what's important, dictating how we feel at every moment of every day. The destination? Well, it's best summed up in a great work of literature, "Ithaca," by the Greek poet Constantine P. Cavafy (1911), about his journey to Ithaca, a mystical place of untold treasures:

Always keep Ithaca in your mind.
To arrive there is your ultimate goal.
But do not hurry the voyage at all.
It is better to let it last for many years;
and to anchor at the island when you are old,
rich with all you have gained on the way,
not expecting that Ithaca will offer you riches.

Ithaca has given you the beautiful voyage.
Without her you would have never set out on the road.
She has nothing more to give you.

And if you find her poor, Ithaca has not deceived you.
Wise as you have become, with so much experience,
you must already have understood what Ithacas mean."

You are on the road to halting, then turning back, the aging process. To get to this place, all you have to do is begin the journey. It's never too late to start. Remember: It's about how young you feel, not how old you actually are. When I am asked my age, I say, "I may be 50 years old to you, but to me, I am 30 and holding."

You can turn back the clock.

Stay true to yourself, think positive, and go at your own pace, but keep going.

Stay in the moment. Enjoy the journey.

You are on your way to a wondrous place.

ACKNOWLEDGMENTS

Writing this book has been quite a growth experience or, in yoga terms, a deep breath, a stretch. But it was possible only because of many people.

First and foremost, Jan Miller and Michael Broussard, my literary agents, at Dupree Miller and Associates. Jan and Michael stepped into my yoga class one night, and immediately after class I was in their office and we were negotiating a book deal.

Thank you, Jan. I have such love and deep appreciation for your absolute, nonstop support and enthusiasm. I honor your total belief in me and treasure your caring and devoted friendship in every way. I cherish you and thank you for everything.

Thank you, Michael. I have such love and deep appreciation for you, your sensitivity, your good humor, and your total belief in me and the yoga program, including the nutritional aspects, which you've been so good in following. You went far beyond your duties as an agent. I appreciate you and cherish our friendship.

To Kurt Twining, my love, my sweetie, my most wonderful husband of only a few months. Thank you for your love, support, and patience. Your sensitivity, truthfulness, and life values have had such a huge impact on me, and those values have been projected through this book and my teaching. Being a technical and computer nerd, thank you for your good humor every time I "lost the file" and you had to drive back from the ranch to "find it."

Thank you to my two precious daughters, Bodine Wolchuk and Kerry Ann Mattolsolio King, for the love the three of us share in our own "Ya Ya sisterhood." Through the thick and thin of life, we share it all. Your never-ending support and encouragement have always been just a minute away. And to Casey Mattosolio King, my son-in-law, thank you for your love and support.

Thank you to Rockport Publishers and associated company Fair Winds Press, for your wonderful hospitality in Gloucester. The photo shoot was a wonderful experience. To all of you who worked on the book, thank you. And a special thanks to Ken Fund, CEO. Thank you, Ken for your hospitality and fabulous tour of Gloucester. Appreciation and thanks to Holly Schmidt, Paula Munier, Silke Braun, Dalyn Miller, Jeff Theis, Wendy Simard, Janelle Randazza, and Regina Grenier.

Silke, a special thanks to you for all your hard work and kind hospitality.

To Mark Seal, thank you for your expertise and professional input on the writing of this book, and for finding the time and energy to complete this project, especially during your bereavement period for the loss of your father. Thank you for your patience and gracefulness when so many times I e-mailed you a file five times, or just one that you couldn't open at all. You are a sweetheart.

To Wendy Graham, thank you for your immediate attention and assistance when the book deal was confirmed. Your help contributed largely to the overall project. You have a beautiful presence, and it is always wonderful having you in yoga whenever you come to Dallas.

To world-class photographer Bobbi Bush and your assistants: Your creativeness and expertise during the photo shoot made it so easy. Thank you for the beautiful photos and your smiling face, even when you were 2 feet deep in water with your tripod.

To Deborah Coull and Lesley Griffin from Deborah Coull Salon and Aveda Concept and Sanctuary Salon: Thank you both for the beautiful makeover, hairstyling, and products.

A special thank you to all my students at the Cooper Aerobics Center and at Larry North Studio, and to all my private clients who witnessed the growth of my practice, my marriage, and this book with so much enthusiasm.

A special thank you to Larry North and your beautiful wife, Melanie, for taking me in as one of the family in your world of fitness. Thank you, Brenda Gillies, for your friendship and for the value you placed on my teachings that brought "my yoga" to Larry North.

To Baron Baptiste, it was a pleasure assisting you in the Yucatan with your yoga retreats. It was a real growing experience for me in many ways. Thank you for your friendship and your expertise. I will always honor and treasure the time we spent together and everything you taught me.

To Houston Institute, where it all began and where I became a certified yoga instructor.

Thank you to a dear friend, Verne Varona. I organized many seminars for your nutritional classes in Dallas, including Parker's Chiropractor's College, and always learned so much from your wisdom.

To Randi Schwartz, my student and friend, you have finally reached your goals. Your committed attendance to yoga classes has taken you to your goal weight and helped you with health issues. I appreciate your great friendship and your support and belief in me, not to mention the beautiful dress you selected for my wedding and the yoga outfits you chose for this book.

To Cory and Ryan Twining, for your patience and guidance, and for the good laugh you had every time the computer went crazy on me. Thank you for your technical expertise and all of your support. I am so grateful to have you in our family. Taylor Twining, thank you for your support; I appreciate you coming to class despite not knowing what it was all about, and giving me that chance.

To Jason Voinov, thank you for your professional and great photos that were originally sent to Fair Winds with the book proposal.

To Mom and Dad, Ann and Hyman Schneider, with love and deep affection. You strove with me to find and follow my dreams through the hard times. Mom and Dad, you were always concerned about my future and how, at the age of 50, I would ever find both a career and a loving and devoted husband to spend the rest of my life with. Well, can you believe it? I found both. I love you two. You are all about what graceful, positive, and youthful aging is all about.

To my sister, Laura Diane Kurlansky, and family. Thank you for your loving support, always, your friendship, and the bond we share. I will get you into yoga, one day. Too many miles separate us, which I hope to shorten soon. My first book goes to you.

To Mom and Dad, Vera and Lew Twining, and the rest of all the Twinings, thank you for your love and support. Vera, you were inspired and took the plunge into yoga classes in your retirement city in Phoenix. I am inspired by you.

To Kathryn Tracy. Thank you for your support from the time I started teaching, following me all around Dallas, traveling an hour to and from yoga to get in your sessions, and for keeping me up to date with my calendar and all my yoga computer needs. You are a gem. I appreciate your thoughtfulness and our beautiful friendship.

And to all of you who are ready to stop and then reverse the aging clock, thank you for stepping onto this road where I have found such treasures and so much love.

ABOUT THE AUTHOR

Glenda Twining received her yoga certification from the Houston Institute and has her Physical Fitness Degree from the Cooper Institute for Aerobics Research. She has studied with acclaimed teachers and gurus, both in the U.S. and abroad—including Baron Baptiste, with whom she ran yoga retreats in the Yucatan. Her philosophy is based on Eastern and Western methods and practices. The inspiration behind her teaching is to provide a balanced workout: A physiologically based fitness regime that promotes increased flexibility, cardiovascular, and body-strengthening results.

Currently, Glenda facilitates classes for health clubs, professional sport teams, and private enthusiasts. Glenda has worked for many years with professional mountain climbers, getting them physically fit for the endurance of their goals, and she also works with overweight individuals getting them to reach their goals.

Glenda is South African and moved to Dallas twenty years ago. She has two grown daughters and is newly married. She splits her time between Dallas and her husband's Cypress Springs Lake ranch in East Texas.